A Psychoanalytic Approach to Smoking Cessation

A Psychoanalytic Approach to Smoking Cessation: The Cigarette as a Transitional Object provides an accessible understanding to the unconscious motive behind smoking addiction using Winnicott's concept of the transitional object.

The book is divided thematically into six parts. Ko begins by outlining the conscious motives for smoking from a psychological perspective and looks at commercial research conducted by the tobacco industry, before using psychoanalytically informed cross-disciplinary literature to assess the unconscious motives for smoking. She expertly introduces Winnicott's view on smoking addiction, using his concept of the transitional object, and highlights the power of the Free Association Narrative Interview method in accessing the unconscious and embedded emotional experiences. Using clinical examples, she illustrates the benefits of this method as a tool to elicit free associations from research respondents. She details the parallels between the individual respondents' smoking experience, as well as their relationship with cigarettes and the seven qualities of transitional objects outlined by Winnicott in his 1953 landmark paper. Ko concludes by emphasising the significance and implications of this thesis to smokers and public health policy, as well as the smoking cessation approach and proposed directions for future research.

This book is an essential resource for psychoanalysts and psychotherapists working in smoking cessation organisations, as well as those working in addiction services.

Fung Ko holds a PhD in Psychoanalytic Studies from the University of Essex, UK. She has 30 years of experience in multinational consumer goods companies marketing 'pleasure food'. Her psychoanalytic research focuses on Winnicott's concept of the transitional object to give understanding to tobacco addiction.

A Psychoanalytic Approach to Smoking Cessation

The Cigarette as a Transitional Object

Fung Ko

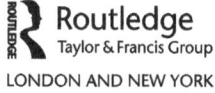

Routledge
Taylor & Francis Group

LONDON AND NEW YORK

Cover image by Frances M. Y. Leung

First published 2024
by Routledge
4 Park Square, Milton Park, Abingdon, Oxon OX14 4RN

and by Routledge
605 Third Avenue, New York, NY 10158

Routledge is an imprint of the Taylor & Francis Group, an informa business

© 2024 Fung Ko

British Library Cataloguing-in-Publication Data
A catalogue record for this book is available from the British Library

Library of Congress Cataloging-in-Publication Data
Names: Ko, Fung, author.
Title: A psychoanalytic approach to smoking cessation : the
cigarette as a transitional object / Fung Ko.
Description: Abingdon, Oxon ; New York, NY : Routledge, 2024. |
Includes bibliographical references and index. |
Identifiers: LCCN 2023027050 (print) | LCCN 2023027051
(ebook) | ISBN 9781032358673 (hardback) | ISBN 9781032354156
(paperback) | ISBN 9781003329077 (ebook)
Subjects: LCSH: Smoking cessation. | Psychoanalysis. |
Nicotine addiction—Treatment.
Classification: LCC RC567 .K58 2024 (print) | LCC RC567 (ebook) |
DDC 616.86/5—dc23/eng/20230817
LC record available at https://lccn.loc.gov/2023027050
LC ebook record available at https://lccn.loc.gov/2023027051

ISBN: 978-1-032-35867-3 (hbk)
ISBN: 978-1-032-35415-6 (pbk)
ISBN: 978-1-003-32907-7 (ebk)

DOI: 10.4324/9781003329077

Typeset in Times New Roman
by codeMantra

For Frances, who stands by me rain or shine, and patiently endures my eccentricity and occasional breakdowns.

Contents

Part IV
**Which research approach has the power to access
the unconscious?**   79

Part V
**The shadow of the transitional object fell
upon the cigarette**   97

Part VI
So what?   141

About the author

Fung Ko is a marketing professional with 30 years of experience marketing 'pleasure food' with highly addictive ingredients: namely caffeine and nicotine. After all these years, she has not become addicted to the product itself, instead she has become more and more interested in the reasons for such a powerful and irrational addiction, and has turned to psychoanalysis for an answer. Since then, she has fallen helplessly in love with psychoanalysis.

At one point in her life, she became very curious about why she was doing what she was doing every day, and how little she could make sense of her own behaviours. Therefore, after getting her bachelor and Master of Business Administration degrees in Hong Kong, she started studying academic psychology on a part-time basis receiving a bachelor's and master's degree respectively while working full-time as a marketing manager at a large multinational tobacco company.

Dissatisfied with the theory of human behaviours based on a conscious level of functioning offered by academic psychology, she found psychoanalysis and the study of the dynamic unconscious. In 2010, she was accepted on the PhD programme at the University of Essex with Professor R. D. Hinshelwood as her research supervisor. During the explorations of the topics of her thesis, she found herself drawn to Winnicott's theory of the mother-infant relationship and his concept of the 'transitional object'. Finally, she landed on the following subject: To what extent can a cigarette be regarded as a regressed form of 'infantile transitional object' that prolongs into adulthood?

Fung Ko received her Doctorate from the University of Essex in 2018 and this book is adapted from her PhD thesis, with Professor R. D. Hinshelwood as the background advisor.

Foreword

This new book by Dr Fung Ko offers a dynamic approach to the subject of cigarette smoking addiction, and how to tackle it. Smoking remains a worldwide addictive habit for all levels of society, rich or poor, young or old, where there is sufficient advertising and/or cultural acceptance.

Dr Ko asks a pertinent question of the reader on this serious and important matter: 'Why has there been little or no scholarly research done on the worldwide human propensity for smoking addiction, without recourse to the significant exploration and understanding of the unconscious factors that may lie at its core?'

Dr Ko first began to consider this question, following on from her own post graduate doctoral study into cigarette addiction, where she proposed the following hypothesis: To what extent can a cigarette be regarded as a regressed form of 'infantile transitional object' that prolongs into adulthood?

Trying to understand cigarette addiction from a psychoanalytic perspective, and largely drawing on the work of Dr D. W. Winnicott and his theory of transitional phenomena in particular, Dr Ko makes a case in this highly readable book for more systematic and widespread clinical trials to take place, following on from these initial beginnings.

Dr Ko elaborates on this significant change of direction in research – that of working with the unconscious – as opposed to solely the rational approach to cigarette addiction, showing how this might be instrumental to further progress in such a difficult field.

Chapter by chapter, the book carefully takes us through several stages, thoroughly exploring the effect of the many research trials undertaken by those involved in marketing this area of tobacco use. It reveals the relative lack of progress that working with standard formulae and hypotheses have produced, largely failing to curb this 'illogical' and dangerous substance abuse.

A reader unfamiliar with the work of the psychoanalyst and paediatrician Donald Winnicott might perhaps wonder at the suggested correlation of Winnicott's Transitional Object with the cigarette, the transitional object being the early attachment object in the life of a young child, the cigarette being seen as a similar, but a more regressed, and pathological attachment. However, Dr Ko's excellent and comprehensive account of Winnicott's general theories of psychoanalysis, and in particular, the relevance of this most well-known of his theoretical papers, gives the reader a clear context for her thinking, and for her choice of this special area to explore.

In a small trial study, Dr Ko suggests how much a recurring theme for the young smokers interviewed was that smoking allowed them to be in a place where there was 'time for me' and for 'relaxation' from cares and responsibilities. In Winnicottian terms this may be seen as the earliest stage of transitional object phenomena, when baby and mother might, as yet, be 'merged', and the infant is carried by 'another' as it were. For the infant, in times of anxiety or need of comfort, such a place is found through the sensory attachment to the given object or repetitive activity (the transitional phenomenon), which, for the infant, is symbolic of the early infant-mother dyad. In normal health this develops, or transitions into separation and individuation for the infant, but in a more pathological version the infant stays 'cocooned' as it were from demands, dependent on the mother. This early behaviour is what is correlated, Dr Ko suggests, with the imagined 'cigarette smoking haven'—a place that is timeless and free from pressures and cares, and where the sensory attachment to the cigarette, and sucking and imbibing and breathing out a substance is akin to a return to maternal closeness, physicality and warmth. It is a regressive and destructive, and perhaps perverse return to a cul-de-sac, inimical to normal healthy development, and perhaps, in unconscious terms, a feature of much addictive behaviour.

The case is skilfully made from this first small clinical trial Dr Ko undertook with young people and their attitudes to their smoking habituation. From thus looking at Winnicottian theory as her resource, she posits that research into unconscious behaviour with respect to cigarette addiction needs to have a much bigger place.

Whilst acknowledging the narcotic effects of the contents of a cigarette, she concludes that what the young smokers do *not* consciously know, or try to evade and suppress, regarding their addiction, needs further time and space for elucidation. Her book indicates that more trials purposely designed to elicit data from this area of unconscious understanding need to go forward to substantiate such a hypothesis.

For the general reader struggling with smoking addiction, to the many researchers in this complex field, Dr Ko's book offers a step change, and hope for thinking about and treating this complex phenomenon.

Helen Taylor Robinson
Joint General Editor with Dr Lesley Caldwell of *The Collected Works of D. W. Winnicott in 12 Volumes* (Oxford University Press, 2016)
Fellow of Institute of Psychoanalysis, UK, Child and Adult Analyst (Retired)

Acknowledgements

From zero knowledge in psychoanalysis to a PhD thesis, and then to this publication project, I am deeply indebted to Professor R. D. Hinshelwood. Not only has he given his selfless support for my academic attainment, he has also given me a fatherly attention that goes beyond merely the intellectual, reminding me to 'stay real' and connected with the clinical aspects of psychoanalysis. Through and through, Bob has been the grandmaster to me. Academic pursuit and the writing quest is a lonely journey, but I have never felt alone.

Introduction

On 12 July 1957, the then United States Surgeon General Leroy Edgar Burney issued an official statement establishing a causal relationship between smoking and lung cancer as a result of a group study by the Advisory Committee on Smoking and Health. Burney declared that 'The Public Health Service feels the weight of the evidence is increasingly pointing in one direction: that excessive smoking is one of the causative factors in lung cancer ... cigarette smoking particularly is associated with an increased chance of developing lung cancer' (United States Department of Health, Education, and Welfare: Public Health Service, 1964, p. 7), and this marked the first reliable large-scale research conducted on the link between smoking and health risk. Since then, there have been multiple studies conducted by different countries confirming the Surgeon General's statement on the risk of smoking, especially cigarette smoking which has been the predominant type of tobacco product (other than cigar, pipe tobacco, chewing tobacco, snus and shisha) used by the general public. The tobacco industry reacted by launching allegedly 'reduced risk' products such as filter, low-tar, and slim cigarettes, but that did not stop governments from implementing various types of tobacco control measures aimed at reducing the smoking prevalence.

According to the World Health Organization (2022), there are 1.3 billion adult smokers globally, this means that one in five adults are smokers. Tobacco is regarded as the most dangerous consumer product and it is estimated that eight million people die from tobacco use each year, including seven million smokers from direct tobacco use and 1.2 million non-smokers from indirect exposure to second-hand smoke (passive smoking).

In an attempt to reduce smoking prevalence, a growing number of countries have tobacco control policies in place: as of 2020, 110 countries have implemented different levels of tobacco control policies, including smoke-free environments legislation, smoking cessation programmes, health warning labels on cigarette packaging, mass media campaign bans, advertising bans, as well as taxation on tobacco products. However, in spite of efforts by governments and the known health risk of smoking, people still continue to smoke. It is predicted that the adult smoking population will remain at 1.3 billion by 2025 (World Health Organization, 2021).

DOI: 10.4324/9781003329077-1

It has been almost 70 years since the publication of the Surgeon General's report, and the causal link between smoking and lung cancer established. However, despite a conscious awareness of its toxic content, people still continue to smoke. Even Freud could not resist a strong addiction to cigars. Having been diagnosed with oral cancer in 1923 at the age of 67, and subsequently, having endured 33 painful operations in the remaining 16 years of his life, he continued to smoke until his death, fully aware that smoking would eventually kill him.

Why do people continue to smoke despite a conscious awareness of tobacco's toxicity? How can we account for the paradox that even educated and intelligent people, who are well aware of the risk of smoking, still continue to take unacceptable health risks – that they are illogically addicted, in effect? I am interested in pursuing the unconscious motivations and reasons for such an illogical and health-risking addiction; this is the area where psychoanalysis can add value to the understanding of smoking addiction, and shed light on the unconscious motive for smoking.

Since this is a book looking at the value of Winnicott's transitional object as a concept to understand smoking addiction, the perspectives of Freud's sexual phantasies and Klein's introjection (inhaling) of internal objects are beyond the scope of this book, they will be mentioned briefly but will not be used to explicate the major thesis. The focus of our research will be in demonstrating the extent to which a cigarette resembles a regressed form of an infantile 'transitional object', a soft object to which an infant becomes attached and that is invested with heightened significance (aka Linus's security blanket), which is prolonged into adulthood, and how the relationship between the smoker and the cigarette resembles that between the infant and the transitional object.

This book is divided into six parts:

Part I: What are the conscious motives for smoking?

We will be looking at the conscious motives for smoking from the perspective of academic psychology and commercial research conducted by the tobacco industry.

Part II: What are the unconscious motives for smoking?

We will examine the unconscious motives for smoking, which is where psychoanalytic investigation of addiction and smoking addiction comes in, including the perspectives from Motivation Research founded by Ernest Dichter, which was the first systematic attempt to apply psychoanalysis to market research, followed by the key development of psychoanalytic understanding on smoking addiction, as well as the psychoanalytically informed cross-disciplinary perspectives on smoking addiction including the views of Edward Bernays, Freud's nephew and regarded as the 'father of public relations', and Isabel Menzies Lyth of the Tavistock Institute of Human Relations.

Part III: What does smoking addiction have to do with Linus's security blanket?

Of all the psychoanalytic theorists within the British Object Relations school, which is the primary theoretical tradition covered in this book, D. W. Winnicott has provided a unique perspective by proposing the idea of transitional object. In his 1953 landmark paper 'Transitional objects and transitional phenomena – a study of the first not-me possession' he observed that between the ages of four and twelve months, children would often become attached to a particular object that they invested with a magical significance. Winnicott called this special item 'the transitional object'; it was the infant's first possession, typically something soft and pliable, readily available and within easy reach of the baby, for example, a piece of wool pulled off a blanket, or a napkin, a teddy bear, or part of a plush toy which a baby clutches and to which it attributes a special value. It is demanded when the infant is about to go to sleep, or at times of stress when the object may be pressed against the infant's face and lips or sucked. When the infant is able to walk, it insists on taking it everywhere. The object retains the smell of the infant and the mother, and therefore it must not be washed, if the object is misplaced, taken away, or lost the infant experiences extreme distress. A well-known example of the transitional object is Linus's security blanket featured in the Peanuts comic strip; coincidentally, Winnicott wrote a letter to the creator of the comic strip, Charles Schulz, seeking permission to reproduce an image of Linus sucking his thumb while clinging to his security blanket for his own book relating to the theory of the transitional object (Winnicott, 1955b).

To Winnicott, a transitional object may be seen as the illusion of a mother substitute for the infant in order to deal with separation anxiety and the loss of omnipotence. The presence of an infantile transitional object represents the existence of an intermediate space of reunion with the mother in the phantasy, and it is 'one of the bridges that make contact possible between the individual psyche and external reality' (Winnicott, 1955a, p. 218). It also constitutes the basis of initiation of experience and object relations of the infant, therefore it is a sign of healthy development. In adulthood, the transitional object loses its meaning, and it gradually widens out over time in the intense experience of the areas of arts, religions, imaginative living and creative scientific work. In his landmark paper of 1953, Winnicott suggested that 'addiction can be stated in terms of regression to the earliest stage at which the transitional phenomena are unchallenged' (Winnicott, 1953, p. 97). We will be using Winnicott's concepts of regression of the transitional phenomena in the understanding of smoking addiction.

Part IV: Which research approach has the power to access the unconscious?

Here, a summary is given on why the Free Association Narrative Interview method (Hollway & Jefferson, 2013) has been chosen as the primary data collection method, instead of more conventional quantitative survey-based and qualitative interview-based research approaches, and explains its power to access the unconscious and embedded emotional experiences through eliciting free associations from the respondents.

Part V: The shadow of the transitional object fell upon the cigarette

In this section a summary of eight respondents' unique personal stories and their relationship with smoking from 16 one-hour interviews using the Free Association Narrative Interview method is presented. Specifically, we will take a closer look at how the respondents' smoking experience and their relationship with cigarettes resembles the seven qualities of transitional object outlined by Winnicott (1953) and the tobacco industry's research on smoking moments will also be used to provide a supplementary framework of analysis to identify the 'regressive' smoking moments.

Part VI: So what?

In Part VI, the contribution of this thesis to the idea of transitional phenomena and cigarette addiction is presented in detail, showing its significance and implications for smokers and public health policy, as well as proposed directions for future research.

Part I

What are the conscious motives for smoking?

In the first chapter, we will be looking at the conscious motives for smoking from the psychological literature and provide an evaluation of these psychological theories of smoking addiction from three dimensions: first, their consideration of the unconscious irrational motives of human behaviours, second, the extent to which the individual assumes a personal agency in their decisions, and finally socio-cultural factors as a significant force in driving addictive behaviours. In conclusion it will be seen that none of the psychological theories provide an adequate consideration of the above three dimensions.

The psychoanalytic approach, on the other hand, may be able to address the inadequacies of the psychological approach and provide a unique and valuable perspective in the understanding of smoking addiction, given its emphasis on the experiential aspect of human behaviours and motivations, as well as allowing a place for the unconscious, which is the perspective taken in this book.

In the second chapter, an overview of a tobacco company's commercial research on 'smoking moments' is given to augment our investigation on 'regressive' smoking moments.

DOI: 10.4324/9781003329077-2

Chapter 1

What do the psychologists think?

I will provide the dictionary definition of addiction and, using information from the World Health Organization, proceed to summarise the seven types of psychological theories of addiction, mapping their evolution from isolated individual theories to integrated and synthetic theories of addiction at both the individual, as well as population and social, levels.

Key sections

- Addiction as a rational choice
- Addiction as an irrational choice
- Addiction as an impulse
- Addiction as a habit acquired through associative learning
- The diffusion of addiction in population
- Integrated theories of addiction
- A synthetic theory of addiction

Despite the known health risk of cigarette smoking, smoking incidence continues to increase: according to the World Health Organization (2022), tobacco is regarded as the most dangerous consumer product that kills the highest number of people. While 0.1 billion people died from tobacco use in the 20th century, it is projected that one billion will die in the 21st century. It is widely known that tobacco contains toxic ingredients; however, what makes it addictive is not the toxic agent itself, but the craving of it, despite conscious awareness of toxicity.

According to the *Oxford Learner's Dictionary* (Oxford University Press, n.d.), addiction means 'the condition of being addicted to something', and 'addicted' means being 'unable to stop taking harmful drugs or using or doing something as a habit', so there is a compulsive dependence element in the dictionary explanation of addiction.

The origin of the word 'addiction' comes from *addictus* in Latin, which means 'to devote, consecrate; sacrifice, sell out, betray, abandon' (Harper, 2022). The

DOI: 10.4324/9781003329077-3

ancient Roman myth tells the story of a debt slave called Addictus who was kept in chains by his master for many years. Even after his debt was paid and he was released by his master, Addictus had become so accustomed to his painful bondage that he could not remove the chains and continued to wander the land with them for the rest of his life, even though they could have been removed at any time (Malinowska, 2018).

A modern and comprehensive definition of addiction is provided by the World Health Organization (2010):

> ... repeated use of a psychoactive substance or substances, to the extent that the user (referred to as an addict) is periodically or chronically intoxicated, shows a compulsion to take the preferred substance (or substances), has great difficulty in voluntarily ceasing or modifying substance use, and exhibits determination to obtain psychoactive substances by almost any means. Typically, tolerance is prominent and a withdrawal syndrome frequently occurs when substance use is interrupted. The life of the addict may be dominated by substance use to the virtual exclusion of all other activities and responsibilities. The term addiction also conveys the sense that such substance use has a detrimental effect on society, as well as on the individual; ... Addiction is a term of long-standing and variable usage. It is regarded by many as a discrete disease entity, a debilitating disorder rooted in the pharmacological effects of the drug, which is remorselessly progressive. From the 1920s to the 1960s attempts were made to differentiate between addiction; and 'habituation', a less severe form of psychological adaptation. In the 1960s the World Health Organization recommended that both terms be abandoned in favour of dependence, which can exist in various degrees of severity ...

From the above definition, addiction involves a progressive dosage, compulsive dependence, difficulty in voluntary cessation and the appearance of withdrawal syndrome after cessation.

From a pharmacological perspective, the addictive quality of tobacco comes from the nicotine compound found naturally in tobacco leaves. Nicotine is a stimulant and when inhaled by means of a cigarette it enters the blood stream and travels to the brain, raising the levels of a neurotransmitter called dopamine, which in turn, produces feelings of pleasure and reward. These neurotransmitters are normally used by the brain to reinforce positive behaviours, such as acquiring food or succeeding in social interactions. Over time, the smoker's brain gets used to the regular nicotine stimulation and requires a similar level of activation in order to function normally.

Pharmacological drivers for addiction are beyond the scope of this book; instead, what we are concerned to understand here are the psychological motives for smoking, first at the conscious level and then at the unconscious level. Our objective here, therefore, is to understand what has already been written about the conscious motives for smoking addiction within the field of academic psychology, and then identify areas that unconscious motives, provided by psychoanalytic theories, can add value to the understanding of the aetiology of addiction.

In summary, psychological theories of addiction can be categorised into six groups: rational choice theories, irrational choice theories, theories focusing on compulsion and self-control, theories emphasising habituation through associative learning, theories focusing on the diffusion of addiction at the population level, and integrated theories of addiction. However, some of these theories are only minor, semantic variations of the others, and they provide only a partial explanation of addiction. For this reason, psychological theories of addiction have made little progress in the past 40 years.

In view of the above inadequacies, West (2006) has proposed a synthetic theory of addiction that attempts to encapsulate different theories which offer unique insights on the psychology of addiction and provide a unifying construct that is capable of generating new ideas moving forward. This is a good start towards a more unifying psychological theory of addiction, although the synthetic theory will need to gain more widespread support before it can become a paradigm psychological theory of addiction (Kuhn, 1962).

In the following paragraphs, we will focus on the specific aspect of addiction that each psychological theory attempts to tackle, and areas that they fail to explain. We will also provide a more detailed description of the synthetic theory of addiction (West, 2006), in order to summarise how the psychological theories of addiction have taken us so far on the journey to understanding the conscious motives of addiction since the 1970s. Finally, the chapter concludes with a critique of each of the psychological theories of addiction in terms of the following: the extent to which they take into consideration the unconscious aspect of attitudes, behaviours and motivation, the place for the individual as an agent in his own decision-making, as well as the socio-cultural factors that influence smoking addiction, and how psychoanalysis can contribute to the understanding of the unconscious motives of addiction.

Addiction as a rational choice

Rational choice theories belong to the economic theory of addiction that viewed addiction as a rational decision-making process aiming at maximising total utility based on a cost-and-benefit analysis.

There were three main theories in this category:

1. The **opponent process theory** suggested that addiction was motivated by the avoidance of distress despite the withdrawal syndrome and the lack of pleasure (Solomon & Corbit, 1973; Solomon, 1980).
2. The **theory of rational addiction** indicated that addictive patterns of behaviours were triggered by stressful life events, and the

addiction worked towards enhancing the overall wellbeing of the addicts (Becker & Murphy, 1988).

3. The **self-medication model of addiction** postulated that addicts intentionally used drugs as a form of self-medication to cope with their own psychological disorders, as well as to regulate their own vulnerabilities such as difficulties in regulating affects, self-esteems, relationships and self-care (Khantzian, 1997; Farrell et al., 2001; Gelkopf et al., 2002).

The rational choice theories offered an incomplete explanation of addiction: it is unlikely that all human decisions are based on a thorough cost-and-benefit analysis as suggested by the opponent process theory, avoidance of distress seems unlikely to be the only cause of loss of control of addictive behaviour as predicted by the opponent process theory, and psychological disorders do not always predate drug use as hypothesised by the self-medication model of addiction. More importantly, rational choice theories failed to account for the fact that many addicts genuinely choose to exercise restraint, wanting to stop, and yet still fail.

Addiction as an irrational choice

Contrary to the assumptions in the rational choice theories that addicts make rational choices, the irrational choice theories suggested that addiction involved an irrational choice that overvalued the benefits and/or undervalued the costs of the addictive behaviours, and this was mainly driven by biases, personal feelings associated with the behaviours and their outcomes, preference for the present over the future, habituation, sensitisation or physiological changes which further strengthened the addictive behaviours.

There were eight prevalent theories in this category:

1. **Expectancy theories** suggested that addiction was driven by the very personal expectations the addicts held regarding the costs and benefits of the addictive activities, regardless of the validity of the expectations (Christiansen & Goldman, 1983; Rather et al., 1992; Tate et al., 1994; Goldman & Darkes, 2004).

2. The **transtheoretical model** argued that recovery from addiction involved a six-stage progression from 'pre-contemplation' in which no change was intended, to 'contemplation' in which change was considered in the next six months, to 'preparation' in which plans

were made for action to be taken in the next month, to 'action' in which the attempt to change were actually made, to 'maintenance' whereby the new behaviour was maintained to prevent relapse, and finally to 'termination' in which the new behaviour was firmly established. Any individual would move back and forth across the six stages and intervention programmes would be tailored according to the addicts' current stage of recovery (Prochaska & Goldstein, 1991; Prochaska, et al., 1985; Prochaska & Velicer, 1997).

3. The **behavioural economics theory** attempted to provide an explanation of addiction using the demand and supply curves in macro-economic theories: the level of addiction could be viewed as a change in the relationship between unit price (the y axis) and consumption quantity (the x axis). As such, an escalation from casual use to an addictive usage pattern could be represented by a shift in the demand curve to the right, and a higher level of addiction could be represented by a steeper demand curve (Jones, 1989; Lewit, 1989; Madden et al., 1997; Madden et al., 1999; Bickel & Marsch, 2001; Dixon et al., 2003; Audrain-McGovern et al., 2004).

4. The **gateway theory** was based on the economic theory that individuals would choose drugs that had the lowest marginal cost and the highest marginal utility, and that addiction to a milder, less powerful drug would predispose one to be more susceptible to other stronger, more addictive drugs. A possible explanation could be that the milder gateway drug might provide a taste of the reward to the addicts, hence facilitating the progression to a more powerful drug in order to achieve a similar level of reward (Kandel et al., 1992; Lindsay & Rainey, 1997; Kenkel et al., 2001; Beenstock & Rahav, 2002; Chen et al., 2002; Tullis et al., 2003).

5. **Choice theory** assumed that individuals' preferences differed in stability and consistency, and addicts were more unstable in their preferences. So addiction was a result of conflicted choices that changed frequently according to the addicts' preferences at certain moments (Skog, 2000).

6. **Cognitive biased theories** suggested that addiction was sustained by the addicts because they tended to pay more attention to and selectively remember information related to their addictive behaviours (Waters & Feyerabend, 2000; Waters et al., 2003: Bradley et al., 2004).

7. **Identity shifts theory** suggested that accumulated dissatisfaction of self-identity caused by addictive behaviours would lead to a conflict of values, prompting small steps towards behavioural changes and ultimately identity shifts; with increased self-awareness and self-confidence of the addicts, continued and persistent change was possible (Kearney & O'Sullivan, 2003).

8. **Affect heuristic theory** argued that people tended to rely heavily on intuitive, rather than analytical, methods of judging the value of different options. So if addicts felt positively about smoking, they would tend to underestimate its associated risks and overestimate its benefits (Slovic et al., 2006).

The irrational choice theories incorporated the role of biases, feelings, temporal priority, habituation, sensitisation and physiological factors in explaining the motives for addiction. However, subsequent validations of these theories mostly generated mixed results, indicating that there was insufficient evidence to conclude that the named irrational factors actually influenced addictive behaviours.

Addiction as an impulse

In order to account for the addicts' failure to exercise restraint despite a genuine and conscious effort, another group of theories emerged and argued that not all addictive activities involved choice: the concepts of disease, impulses, urges, inhibitory forces, self-control, and voluntary restraint in understanding addiction should be taken in consideration.

A total of seven theories fell into this category:

1. The **disease model of addiction** viewed addiction as a medical disorder caused by structural and functional abnormality in the central nervous system which led to impairment of self-control. So for the addicts, there was no real choice, only compulsion (Edwards & Gross, 1976; Gelkopf et al., 2002).

2. The **abstinence violation effect theory** suggested that probability of relapse would be higher if the addict had a destructive

cognitive process, attributing the cause of his relapse to internal, stable and global attributes (Marlatt, 1979).

3. **Tri-dimensional personality theory** suggested that addicts could be divided into three personality sub-types, including novelty seeking, harm avoidance and reward dependence types. These personality dimensions and their interactions had direct impact on an individual's susceptibility to addiction, leading to different patterns of response to novelty, punishment and rewards, which in turn resulted in different levels of dependence on drug and alcohol (Cloninger, 1987).

4. The **cognitive model of drug urges** suggested that compulsive drug use was a result of highly automated action sequences learned through repetitions, and that desire and intent to drug use were paired in active smokers and unpaired in those who were try quit smoking (Tiffany 1990, 1999; Tiffany & Conklin, 2000).

5. **Self-efficacy theory** proposed that an individual's self-confidence in his ability to achieve certain outcomes was a key determinant in driving behaviour changes, and that a decrease in self-efficacy would trigger and reinforce a sense of loss of control in addiction (Marlatt, 1996; Niaura, 2000; Gwaltney et al., 2001).

6. **Self-regulation theory** postulated that there were individual differences in addicts' propensity to exercise self-control, and these differences in self-regulation ability contributed to the development of addictive behaviours (Baumeister & Heatherton, 1996).

7. **Inhibition dysregulation theory** argued that impaired decision-making ability caused by a dysfunctional inhibitory system or reward system in respective brain regions was responsible for the compulsive behaviours associated with addiction (Lubman et al., 2004).

The impulse theories took into consideration the concept of self-control and compulsion in addiction, however, they failed to provide an explanation for those addictive behaviours which seemed to occur without conscious awareness, as well as for the apparent disconnection between the overpowering urge of the addicts to engage in addictive behaviours and the perceived rewards from drugs.

Addiction as a habit acquired through associative learning

The associative learning theories regarded addiction as a habitual behavioural pattern developed through repetitions that were outside the addict's conscious awareness. The resultant impulses to engage in addictive behaviours could be so powerful that they overwhelmed any desires and effort by the addicts to exercise restraint, despite the lack of pleasure. As such, addiction was not always linked to enjoyment or stress relief.

Six theories fell into this category:

1. The **theory of instrumental learning** suggested that addictive behaviour became engrained in addicts through the operant conditioning process, which involved the part of the brain that trains animals to acquire behaviours that assist with survival and reproduction. Such automated learning processes could occur without the addicts being consciously aware of it; it did not involve a rational cost-and-benefit analysis or an active decision-making process, and it did not require the addicts to experience any pleasure from the addictive behaviours (Lewis, 1990; O'Brien et al., 1992; Schulteis & Koob, 1996).

2. The **classical learning theory** suggested that addiction was driven by repeated pairings of environmental stimuli and drug effects. Escalation from casual drug use to addiction could be explained by a strengthening of the learned, associative link between the stimulus preceding the drug dose and the drug dose proper, which in turn amplified the intensity of internal regulation; the internal regulation that occurred in the absence of the drug dose proper would then induce a state of disequilibrium in the addicts and hence, the withdrawal syndrome (Melchior & Tabakoff, 1984; Childress et al., 1988; Drummond et al., 1990; Azorlosa, 1994; Drummond, 2001; Siegel & Ramos, 2002).

3. The **theory of independent learning systems** was a variation of instrumental and classical learning models that emphasised neural mechanisms of learning and memory. All behavioural changes, including the development of drug addiction, involved the storage of new information in the nervous system through three independent learning systems in the brain. Reinforcers operated on these memory systems in three ways: they activated the neural mechanisms involved in approach or avoidance responses, they produced rewarding or aversive states, and they changed or strengthened the representation of the information stored in these memory systems. Each addictive drug mimicked some or all of these mechanisms in

different ways, these reinforcing actions in turn influenced behaviours by acting on the learning and memory systems (White, 1996).

4. The **incentive sensitisation theory** highlighted how drug cues could trigger excessive motivation for the consumption of the actual drugs, resulting in compulsive drug-seeking, drug-taking and relapse. The theory posited that the intake of an addictive substance would put the brain circuitry into high alert so that further intake would produce a greater effect, and that addiction was caused by increased drug-induced sensitisation in the brain that attributed incentive salience ('wanting') to reward-associated stimuli (drug-associated cues), leading to a pathological 'wanting' for drugs. One important premise of this theory was that the sensitised neural systems responsible for 'wanting' could be dissociated from neural systems responsible for the 'liking' of drugs, which helped account for the weak relationship between level of addictiveness of a particular drug and the amount of pleasure it provided (Robinson & Berridge, 1993, 2003).

5. The **social learning theory** focused on the recovery process and extended the instrumental learning theory by incorporating learning through observation and communication. Social learning theory recognised that different types of drugs would exert different effects on different individuals, and that such individual differences were driven by their personality traits and social environment such as their past history and current life circumstances. The theory also emphasised the impact of the addicts' personal 'resources' on their abilities to deal with lapse and relapse (Bandura et al., 1977).

6. The **theory of different drug effects** argued that addiction was the result of the interplay between the stimulation of the dopamine projections to the shell and the core of the nucleus accumbens. Increased extra-synaptic dopamine in the shell of the nucleus accumbens led to pleasurable sensation experienced in smoking, which increased the probability that the activity would be repeated as a result of the operant conditioning mechanism. At the same time, nicotine also caused an increase in dopamine level in the core of the nucleus accumbens and injected 'incentive salience' to cues preceding the drug dose, leading to the onset of the classical conditioning mechanism in the presence of those cues. One differentiating characteristic of nicotine was that the act of smoking, and the cues associated with it, were themselves incentives, this could account for

the observation that the sensory characteristics of smoking such as the smell of tobacco and the sensation in the throat generated by cigarette smoke were sufficient to provide pleasure and satisfaction in the short term (Pritchard et al., 1996; Balfour, 2004).

Learning theories focused on associative learning mechanisms that operated outside of conscious awareness to explain addictive behaviours. Again, they only provided a partial explanation of addiction, and mentalist concepts such as choice, psychological resource, and self-control were still required in order to provide a more comprehensive explanation of addictive behaviours.

The diffusion of addiction in population

Even though the rules underlying group behaviours might not be exactly the same as those underlying individual behaviours, there should be a link between the two, and the observation of group behaviours should, in theory, shed light on the rules governing individual behaviours.

There were two key theories that focused on studying addiction at the population and social group levels:

1. **Diffusion theory** regarded the occurrence of addictive behaviours in populations as a diffusion of uptake or cessation of these behaviours from subgroups to other groups through social networks and geographical proximity. This was consistent with Einstein and Epstein's (1980) findings that 40 per cent of an adult sample smoker group claimed that their smoking initiations were caused by peer influence in a group setting. In addition, the spread of tobacco was regarded as an example of cultural diffusion: the first reported use of tobacco by Europeans was in the late 15th to the early 16th century, and there was a gap of 12 years between reported tobacco use by an English explorer and widespread smoking in England. Furthermore, the popularity of smoking might also be due to the free provision of cigarettes to servicemen during the First and Second World Wars, which resulted in positive, normative and economic reinforcement of cigarette smoking (Einstein & Epstein, 1980; Ferrence, 2001).

2. To account for the development of certain illicit drug use at certain locations and at certain times in certain sub-populations, **trend theory** attributed the key contributors to the distribution system of the illicit drug and the susceptibility of the population as a result of the prevailing political climate (Agar & Reisinger, 2002).

Both diffusion theory and trend theory only focused on some features of addiction and failed to provide a comprehensive explanation of the spread of addiction in populations.

Integrated theories of addiction

There were very few psychological theories that attempted to integrate various factors including rational and irrational choice, self-control, habituation and learning, and the diffusion of addiction in populations into a comprehensive framework of addiction, with the exception of the excessive appetites theory and the model of pathological gambling.

1. The **excessive appetites theory** proposed that addiction could be regarded as an 'appetitive consumption' of particular experiences, it became pathological when the initial pleasure experienced by addicts became out of control, leading to compulsion to engage in addictive activities to the extent that their normal daily activities were intruded upon. Under the excessive appetites theory, escalation from normal consumption to addiction happened via two possible routes: the first route was the 'law of proportionate effect' in which the individuals perceived the incentives of the appetitive activity to be greater than the restraints; this aspect of the theory was intended to capture the choice and self-control elements of addiction. The second route was encapsulated in learning theories involving instrumental and classical conditioning, the consequences of conflicts could be viewed as a tertiary process to further amplify the addiction through demoralisation, poor information processing, and alterations of social role and social group (Orford, 2001).
2. The **pathway model of pathological gambling** postulated that pathological gambling was driven by interactions of ecological, social, psychological and biological factors that generated three primary

pathways and different manifestations of addictive behaviours. The model suggested that there were three subgroups of gamblers, including behaviourally conditioned problem gamblers, emotionally vulnerable problem gamblers and antisocial, and impulsive problem gamblers. Although this model only addressed pathological gambling behaviours, it was also relevant to other addictive behaviours especially in its attempt to integrate decision-making, environmental factors, personality and instrumental learning mechanisms into the model (Blaszcyzynski & Nower, 2002).

Integrated theories of addiction managed to provide a comprehensive account of addiction by recognising the diversity of different factors, patterns, feelings and routes to addiction, as proposed by various specific theories of addiction. However, in order to propel the psychological theory of addiction forward, we need a theory that does more than summarise all the past theories of addiction; the theory needs to provide a unifying framework of addiction that is capable of generating new insights and moving us forward.

To summarise, addiction could be regarded as actions that people take in response to overpowering desires, urges, and impulses in order to engage in certain activities, despite genuine attempts to exercise restraint. There is a sense of loss of control in these addictive activities, and they are not merely an outcome of choices. Choices, be they rational or irrational, are only relevant when individuals consciously weigh the alternatives based on their informed or ill-informed, stable or unstable preferences. In many cases, addicts do not normally consider alternatives and some activities may not even operate on a conscious level. Activities that can be classified as addictive are those where the desires, urges or impulses to engage with them are abnormally powerful, and/or the restraints are abnormally weak. Various factors could influence the initiation, development and maintenance of addiction, including first, the nature of the individuals in terms of their psychological susceptibility, personal traits, beliefs, and values; second, the nature of the activity such as the level of pleasure, satisfaction, or relief from stress it provides; third, the degree to which it taps into instrumental and classic learning mechanisms or leads to neuroadaptation that amplifies both the pleasurable and the punishing effects of the activity; and finally, environmental factors, including opportunities, reminders, cues, situations, and social norms that create needs that could be satisfied by addictive activities.

Building on the various theories of addiction that have been developed so far, West (2006) has proposed a synthetic theory of addiction that does more than summarise various specific theories of addiction, as he also attempts to add value by developing a unifying construct that is capable of generating new ideas in the psychology of addiction.

A synthetic theory of addiction

According to West (2006), addiction is a social construct that involves a chronic condition of the motivational system, in which a disproportionally high priority is given to particular, harmful, reward-seeking behaviours. Addiction can arise from many different abnormalities, so it should be regarded as a symptom rather than a unitary disorder; it varies in severity and has different manifestations as a result of the interactions of personality, social and environmental factors surrounding addicts.

There are three types of pathologies underlying addiction: abnormalities in the motivational system that are not directly caused by addictive behaviours, abnormalities in the motivational system caused by addictive behaviours directly, and pathological environments acting on a normal motivational system that are not equipped to cope with them. All these pathologies have a significant impact on human behaviour.

The synthetic theory of addiction (West, 2006) postulated that the development of addiction is driven by the influence of environmental forces on an inherently unstable motivational system. In this unstable system, environmental forces that create an unbalanced input, or the absence of a balanced input, would send that system down an even more entrenched pathway in the epigenetic landscape, leading to the persistent nature of addictive behaviours.

In view of the multiplicity of factors involved in addiction, psychological theories of addiction have evolved from an abundance of isolated individual theories, each capturing snapshots of some elements of addiction, culminating in West's synthetic theory of addiction (2006), which provides a broad brush of the underlying developmental process and dynamics of addiction. Despite efforts by the synthetic theory of addiction to provide an answer to major questions, such as what activities are addictive, who is susceptible to addiction, what circumstances promote addiction, when and how addiction develops, etc., it still fails to answer the fundamental questions of why there would be individual differences in our motivational system (epigenetic landscape) to start with, and what the factors driving such differences are. Furthermore, the synthetic theory will also need to gain more widespread support before it can become a single paradigm psychological theory of addiction (Kuhn, 1962). All in all, there seems to be no clear winner, and none of the 29 psychological theories described in this chapter can claim to be the truth, though they can claim some of it.

With its emphasis on the cognitive behavioural aspect of human behaviour and motivation, the academic psychological approach in understanding conscious motives of addiction seems to have paid little attention to the unconscious motivations, some of which neglected the role of the individual as an agent in their own decisions, and many mentioned very little about socio-cultural factors as a significant force in driving addictive behaviours. Table 1.1 is a summary of how the psychological theories perform on each of the above three main dimensions:

Table 1 Evaluation of psychological theories of addiction

	Consideration of unconscious motivations	Individual as an agent	Socio-cultural factors as a significant force
1. RATIONAL CHOICE THEORIES			
1.1 Opponent process theory	No	Yes	No
1.2 Theory of rational addiction	No	Yes	No
1.3 Self-medication model	No	Yes	No
2. IRRATIONAL CHOICE THEORIES			
2.1 Expectancy theories	No	Yes	No
2.2 Trans theoretical theories	No	Yes	No
2.3 Behavioural economics theories	No	Yes	No
2.4 Gateway theory	No	Yes	No
2.5 Choice theory	No	Yes	No
2.6 Cognitive bias theories	No	Yes	No
2.7 Identity shifts theory	No	Yes	No
2.8 Affect heuristic theory	No	Yes	No
3. IMPULSE THEORIES			
3.1 Disease model	No	No	No
3.2 The abstinence violation effect	No	No	No
3.3 Tri-dimensional personality theory	No	No	No
3.4 Cognitive model of drug urges	Yes	No	No
3.5 Self-efficacy theory	No	No	No
3.6 Self-regulation theory	No	No	No
3.7 Inhibition dysregulation theory	No	No	No
4. ASSOCIATIVE LEARNING THEORIES			
4.1 Instrumental learning	No	No	No
4.2 Classical learning	No	No	No
4.3 Independent learning systems	No	No	No
4.4 Incentive sensitisation theory	No	No	No
4.5 Social learning theory	No	No	Yes
4.6 Theory of differential drug effects	No	No	No
5. POPULATION LEVEL THEORIES			
5.1 Diffusion theory	No	No	Yes
5.2 Trend theory	No	No	Yes
6. INTEGRATIVE / SYNTHETIC THEORIES			
6.1 Excessive appetites theory	No	Yes	Yes
6.2 Pathways model of pathological gambling	No	Yes	Yes
6.3 Synthetic theory of addiction	No	Yes	Yes

Chapter 2

What do the tobacco boys think?

Since 2013, there have been extensive studies within the tobacco industry on different types of smoking 'moments' in order to gain a better understanding of unmet consumer needs in these moments, and more importantly, to build brand equity and product innovations by linking different brands and offers to specific consumer smoking moments; this is of utmost importance for an industry that is losing social currency and is stigmatised in an increasing number of countries. This research was conducted not just for knowledge but primarily for commercial reasons. In this chapter, we will be analysing commercial research aimed at sales and profit to accumulate knowledge in smoking addiction.

There follows an overview of the findings of research on the smoking moment and 'regressive' moments, from a psychoanalytic perspective, will be identified. This mega-research was fully funded by a commercial tobacco company and is not available in the public domain; the respective insights provided in this chapter have been sourced from 30 years of working in the marketing and consumer insight departments of a tobacco company.

Key ideas

The eight major smoking moments:

1. Pass the time   (Personal moment)
2. Me time   (Personal moment)
3. Self-reward   (Personal moment)
4. Relax   (Personal moment)
5. Focus/problem solver   (Personal moment)
6. Boost/start-up   (Personal moment)
7. Projection of self   (Social moment)
8. Socialise   (Social moment)

DOI: 10.4324/9781003329077-4

As a result of increasing regulations imposed on the tobacco industry, from advertising restrictions in terms of electronic, print and out-of-home media, the application of plain packaging, a ban on retail display and point of sale promotional materials, to consumption restrictions in the form of increasing excise duties and item price, a public place smoking ban and indoor smoking ban, to product restrictions in the form of ingredient restrictions, cigarette stick and pack standardisation, the tobacco industry is rapidly losing its social currency. In the 21st century, the tightening of the regulatory environment together with increasing social stigmatisation of smoking has led to a fundamental change in consumer consumption behaviours from habitual consumption to more conscious and considered consumption. This is characterised by a significant reduction in average daily consumption amounts, from daily regular consumption to consumption only at specific moments; from a high aspirational value of cigarette brand images to that of price-driven commodity, from being able to smoke anywhere, anytime, regardless of others, to choosing to smoke only at a certain time and in certain prescribed places. Traditional smoking behaviour was driven by moments of indulgence, that is, purely pleasure seeking, whereas 21st-century smoking behaviour is driven by moments of enjoyment with a need to balance pleasure with self-responsibility.

In view of changing consumer smoking behaviours, the tobacco industry started investigating different smoking moments, in order to gain a better understanding of the consumer needs driving those moments. A large-scale desktop research was commissioned in order to review cross-category products and understand the type of consumption moments with which these product categories and brands are associated. These product categories included seven focus categories of tea, coffee, beer, spirits, wine and champagne, chocolates, chewing gum and mints, as well as other cross-categories, including aerated and flavoured drinks, energy and functional drinks, cheese, dressings, packaged snacks, frozen foods, fragrance, personal care products, clothes, watches, credit and debit cards, diamonds, greeting cards and cars. The research was conducted in 15 countries including six mature tobacco markets (Japan, South Korea, Australia, Germany, Italy and Canada), eight developing markets (Russia, Ukraine, Turkey, Romania, Malaysia, Brazil, South Africa and Mexico), and one emerging market (Indonesia). The same study also reviewed categories adjacent to tobacco and seeking to identify the type of moods with which these product categories and brands were associated. These product categories included beer, wine and spirits, non-alcoholic beverages, confectionery, food, personal and beauty care across the same 15 countries. In addition, a vigorous approach was undertaken, in order to identify the key moments relevant for the tobacco industry. Another large-scale qualitative research and ethnographic study was conducted by interviewing over 220 consumers; all of them were interviewed three times in order to understand the nuances and depth of their consumption moments using tobacco and also in other categories. In addition, 16 experts were interviewed to further deepen the understanding, and 600 advertisements across eight international markets were analysed within and without the tobacco category to understand each moment's cross-category context, and to explore moments in different regions, cultures and levels of market development.

1. A **cross-category qualitative research** conducted in 15 countries covering markets of different maturity level across seven focus cross-category products including tea, coffee, beer, spirits, wine and champagne, chocolates, chewing gum and mints, in order to understand the type of consumption moments which these product categories and brands are associated with.
2. A large-scale **ethnographic study** with in-depth interviews of over 220 consumers, each with three interviews to cover the nuances and depth of their consumption moments in tobacco and other adjacent product categories.
3. An **expert panel** with 16 experts reviewing and analysing more than 600 advertisements across eight countries to understand each consumption moment's cross-category context and their interactions, and to explore consumption moments of different cultures and levels of market development.

The above studies revealed that there were altogether eight smoking moments relevant to the tobacco industry, each of which is rooted in one core human need underpinning the motivation of their behaviours (see Table 2.1). Of the eight identified smoking moments, the first six related to personal aspects of smoking, and the last two to social aspects of smoking.

1. The '**Pass the time**' smoking moment is driven by a core need to occupy empty moments. The smoker wants to fill empty or dull moments, so there is an absence of stimulation or purpose in this moment. The emotional benefit of the cigarette is to make them feel stimulated and entertained, and the functional benefit of the cigarette is to keep them occupied and busy. The smoking ritual in this moment is characterised by mindless smoking, an average draw of cigarette smoke, rapid inhalation and exhalation, and a low frequency of puffs.
2. The '**Me time**' smoking moment is driven by the smoker's core need to have time alone, which can be further divided into two sub-types: 'time out' and 'time to be myself' moments. In the 'time out' moment, the smoker wants to distinctly isolate themselves to free their mind. The emotional benefit of the cigarette is to keep them out of reach from overstimulation, make them feel free to be themselves, and the functional benefit of the cigarette is to provide them with a short period of isolation. The smoking ritual in this moment is characterised by mindless smoking, a weak draw, inhalation and exhalation, a low frequency of puffs,

and they do not always finish the entire cigarette. In the 'time to be myself' moment, the smoker wants to reclaim themselves through isolation; the emotional benefit of a cigarette is thus, to make them feel free to be themselves, liberated and calm, while the functional benefit of the cigarette is to allow them a significant period of isolation as a kind of escapism. The smoking ritual in the 'time to be myself moment' is characterised by mindless product handling, a weak draw, inhalation and exhalation, and a low frequency of puffs.

3. The '**Self-reward**' smoking moment is driven by the core need for indulgence. The emotional benefit of the cigarette is to make the smoker feel fulfilled, accomplished and proud, as if they deserve something special, and the functional benefit of the cigarette is to give them pleasure and is an indulgence. The smoking ritual in this moment is characterised by a slow pace, deep inhalation and exhalation, and product savouring. Often the smoke is kept in the smoker's mouth for a prolonged duration.

4. The '**Relax**' smoking moment is driven by the core need for self-rebalancing, and it can be further divided into two sub-types of 'revive' and 'de-charge' moments. In the 'revive' moment, the smoker wants to take in positive energy and emotions. The emotional benefit of the cigarette is to make them feel restored and renewed, and the functional benefit of the cigarette is to provide inner balance. The smoking ritual in this moment is characterised by deep inhalation and exhalation, an average-to-weak number of puffs, longer duration in-between puffs, and product savouring. In the 'de-charge' moment, the smoker wants to let go of negative energy and emotions. The emotional benefit of the cigarette is to make them feel as if they have regained control, and the functional benefit of the cigarette is to relieve stress and allow inner balance. The smoking ritual in this moment is characterised by deep inhalation and exhalation, a high frequency of puffs, a short time between puffs, and a tight hand and mouth grip when they smoke.

5. The '**Focus/problem solver**' moment is driven by the core need to concentrate and strengthen the thought process, and it can be further divided into two sub-types of 'focus' and 'problem solver' moments. In the 'focus' moment, the smoker wants to reboot their mind by stepping out. The functional benefit of the cigarette is to help them concentrate and reduce external stimulation, and the emotional benefit of the cigarette is to make them feel creative. The smoking ritual is characterised by an intense draw, infrequent puffs, taking in a lot of smoke, and ignoring ash. In the 'problem solver' moment, the smoker wants to sustain concentration by reducing external irritation. The functional benefit of the cigarette is to provide a mental reboot and gain a clearer mind, and the emotional benefit of the cigarette is to make them feel capable, sharp, and efficient. The smoking ritual is characterised by a strong first draw, infrequent puffs, a superficial inhalation and exhalation, and the cigarette is often left in the ashtray.

6. The '**Boost/start-up**' smoking moment is driven by the need to manage performance and energy levels, and it can be further divided into two sub-types

of 'boost' and 'start-up' moments. In the 'boost' moment, the smoker wants to refuel when their energy levels are low. The functional benefit of the cigarette is to provide an immediate surge of energy, and the emotional benefit of the cigarette is to make them feel capable and strong. The smoking ritual in this moment is characterised by a strong first draw, a high frequency of puffs, no product savouring, exertion of strong pressure on the filter, and intense draws. In the 'start-up' moment, the smoker wants to wake up gently and build motivation. The functional benefit of the cigarette is to provide gradual but long-lasting energy, and the emotional benefit is to make them feel motivated, optimistic and ready. The smoking ritual in this moment is characterised by a weak first draw followed by a weak inhalation and exhalation, a low frequency of puffs; smoke is often retained in the mouth for a prolonged duration.

7. The '**Projection of self**' smoking moment is driven by the core need to control what others see of the smoker, and it can be further divided into two sub-types: 'impress' and 'blend in' moments. The 'impress' moment is when the smoker wants to be noticed and stand out. The functional benefit of the cigarette is to help them stand out, and the emotional benefit of the cigarette is to make them powerful, proud, superior and desirable. The smoking ritual in this moment is characterised by a confident manner, the display of smoking skills, graceful handling of sticks, stick kept in mouth, and play with the cigarette pack or lighter. The 'blend in' moment is when the smoker wants to comply with the codes and norms of the people around them; the emotional benefit of the cigarette is to gain acceptance of like-minded others and to avoid rejection. The functional benefit of the cigarette is to help the smoker blend in and not stand out. The smoking ritual in this moment is characterised by directing smoke away, infrequent puffs, no savouring, and not always smoking the entire cigarette.

8. The '**Socialise**' smoking moment is motivated by the core need to feel close, bond and share with others; the emotional benefit of the cigarette is to enable connection with others, experience light-heartedness, and appreciation by others. The functional benefit of the cigarette is to help with the exchange of ideas and experiences with others, and to provide proximity and connection. The smoking ritual in this moment is characterised by infrequent draws, directing cigarette smoke outwards, and mindless smoking.

The industry study described above also suggests that habitual and routine consumption is not a moment of its own, but rather a weaker version of any of the given moments, which are more habitual and less implicating. The eight smoking moments can be further clustered into four key categories, including 'connection with self'; 'self-balance'; 'performance'; and 'connection with others'. 'Me time' and 'pass the time' moments both satisfy the smokers' need for 'connection with self'; 'self-reward' and 'relax' moments satisfy the smokers' needs for 'self-balance'; 'focus/problem solver' and 'start-up/boost' moments are about achieving 'performance'; 'projection of self', and 'socialise' moments are both about 'connection with others'. All four categories of smoking moments are universal

Table 2.1 Eight major smoking moments

	PERSONAL MOMENTS										SOCIAL MOMENTS		
	CONNECT WITH SELF			SELF BALANCE			PERFOMANCE				CONNECTING WITH OTHERS		
Moments	1a	1b		2a	2b		3a		3b		4a		4b
	Pass the time	Me Time		Self-reward	Relax		Focus/problem solver		Boost/start up		Projection of self		Socialise
Core needs	*Occupy empty momentes*	*Time on my own*		*Indulge myself*	*Rebalancing myself*		*Concentraing and thoght process*		*Manage perfomance and energy levels*		*Control what others see of me*		*Bond and share*
Types	**Pass the time**	**Time to be myself**	**Time out**	**Self-reward**	**De-charge**	**Revive**	**Focus**	**Problem solver**	**Boost**	**Satrt up**	**Impress**	**Blend in**	**Socialise**
Benefits: Functional	Occupied, Busy	Significant period of isolation, escapism	Short period of isolation	Pleasure and indulgence	Stress relief, inner balance	Inner balance	Concentration, reduction of external stimulation	Mental reboot, clearer mind	Immediate surge of energy	Gradual but long-lasting energy	Stand out	Blend in, not stand out	Exchange ideas and things, proximity, connection to others
Benefits: Emotional	Stimulated, entertained	Free to be myself, liberated, calm	Out of reach from over stimulation, free to be myself	Fulfilled, deserving, special, accomplished, proud	Soothed, calmed down, back in control,	Restored, recharged, renewed	Capable, sharp, efficient	Creative	Capable, strong	Motivated, optimistic, ready	Powerful, proud, superior, desirable	Accepted by like-minded others, desirable	Connection with others, light-hearted, appreciated

and can be found in all eight countries surveyed with a varied level of prominence for different moments depending on the level of economic development and the extent of social stigma associated with smoking. For example, 'connection with others' and 'performance' moments are more prominent in emerging markets such as Vietnam and Bangladesh where a cigarette still functions as social currency, whereas 'self-balance' and 'connection with self' moments are more relevant in developed markets such as Canada, Japan, and South Korea, where the awareness level of the risk of smoking is much higher, and where social stigma associated with smoking is also higher. Developing markets such as Brazil, Ukraine, and Turkey present an intermediate situation tending towards the mature market scenarios.

A cigarette is highly versatile and multi-purposed; it has different uses including highly personal functions in terms of building a connection with oneself, fostering self-balance and driving personal performance, and the social type of usage such as connecting with others by cigarette smoking. Our interest is in the individual and personal quality of smoking addiction, not the social aspects of it. This personal quality of smoking is also a highly irrational one, as smokers choose to continue to smoke despite knowing that it will damage their health. If smoking addiction is driven by irrational factors, then what are the unconscious motivations driving such an irrational behaviour? The problem with the 'smoking moments' research from the tobacco industry is that it only addresses conscious experiences and omits the unconscious; it therefore cannot explain the paradox that educated and intelligent people, who are well aware of the risks of smoking still continue to do so – they are, in effect, illogically addicted. We are interested in pursuing unconscious motivation and the reasons for such an illogical and health-risking addiction, and this is the area where psychoanalysis can add value to the understanding of smoking addiction.

Part II

What are the unconscious motives for smoking?

What is puzzling and remains unanswered by psychological theories and the tobacco industry's commercial research focusing on the conscious motives for smoking addiction, is the paradox that educated and intelligent people who are well aware of the risk of smoking still continue to take unacceptable health risks – they are, in effect, illogically addicted. But why?

With its emphasis on the cognitive behavioural aspect of human behaviour and motivation which operates on a conscious level, the academic, psychological approach in understanding addiction seems to have paid little attention to unconscious motivations, some of which neglect the role of the individual as an agent in their own decisions, and mention very little about the socio-cultural factors as a significant force in driving addictive behaviours. The 'smoking moments' research from the tobacco industry was conducted with the sole purpose of driving commercial benefits instead of academic knowledge, therefore it only addresses smokers' conscious experiences in order to make recommendations more concrete and actionable; the problem with that approach is that it omits the unconscious and therefore cannot provide an explanation on the above paradox.

We are interested in pursuing knowledge on unconscious motivation and the reasons for such illogical and health-risking yet powerful addictive behaviour. Given its emphasis on experiential aspects of human behaviours and motivations, as well as allowing a place for the unconscious, the psychoanalytic approach seems to be able to address the inadequacies of the psychological approach and provide a unique and valuable perspective in the understanding of smoking addiction.

However, a PEP-Web search suggests that despite an abundance of literature published on addiction in general, very few papers have been published directly on the subject of smoking. But if we turn to the marketing and social science field as a basis for a search of the literature, we can see evidence of an early influence of psychoanalysis on the understanding of smoking addiction.

In the following chapters, we will first provide an overview of Motivation Research founded by Ernest Dichter in the 1930s. This was the first systematic attempt to apply psychoanalysis to market research and generated some insights on smoking addiction; second, we will look at the key development of psychoanalytic understanding on addictions in general and smoking addiction in particular. Finally,

DOI: 10.4324/9781003329077-5

we will be covering psychoanalytically informed cross-disciplinary perspectives on smoking addiction.

Key sections

- Ernest Dichter's 'Motivation Research'
- Psychoanalytic understanding
- Psychoanalytically informed cross-disciplinary perspectives

Chapter 3

Ernest Dichter's 'Motivation Research'

Smoking is a transcendent pleasure that overpowers any religious, moral and legal reasoning

Due to a general discontent with the failure of conventional quantitative market research to predict consumer behaviours during the 1930s, a group of Austrian émigré psychoanalysts and psychologists, including Paul Lazarsfeld and Ernest Dichter (Horowitz, 1986), attempted to apply psychoanalytic theories to the understanding of the 'why' of consumer behaviours in the marketing and advertising field. A plethora of qualitative consumer research called 'Motivation Research', which utilised various observation and questioning techniques borrowed from clinical psychology, was conducted and published by these social scientists.

In this chapter, we will first provide a general overview on Motivation Research and its evolution, followed by a spotlight on Ernest Dichter – the most controversial figure in Motivation Research. We will also provide an overview of the main findings of Motivation Researchers during the 20 years between the 1930s and the 1950s, when Motivation Research was at its peak, followed by an evaluation of its merits and shortcomings.

What is Motivation Research?

Motivation Research, a name derived from the study of human motives, marked the first systematic attempt made by social scientists to apply psychoanalytic theories and knowledge in the understanding of seemingly irrational consumer behaviours. It was triggered by a general dissatisfaction with a perceived lack of depth and analytic subtlety in conventional quantitative market research and economic thinking in the 1930s, which usually failed to explain the motivations behind consumer behaviours. Contrary to conventional experimental-statistical research which made use of large samples, tabulations and statistics to determine the 'what' and 'how' of consumer behaviours, Motivation Research claimed to focus on the analysis of unconscious wishes, desires, needs and drives, which in turn determined why consumers bought one brand and not another competing alternative, despite having similar functionalities (Williams, 1957).

DOI: 10.4324/9781003329077-6

The underlying assumption of Motivation Research was that when consumers were asked directly about why a certain purchase was made, they either did not know the reason for the purchase, or did not want to disclose the true reason, hence they tended to provide socially acceptable answers. Motivation Researchers suggested that the most important factor influencing consumers' choices were illogical emotions instead of logical reasons, with repressed drives as the most powerful motivators. As such, Motivation Research was developed as a way to tap into the unconscious of consumers to find out the true reasons for purchase (Samuel, 2010). Amongst the various borrowed techniques from the social science disciplines, depth interviews and projective techniques were most widely used by Motivation Researchers.

1. **Depth interviews** involved hours of one-to-one interviews conducted by a Motivation Researcher with no predetermined question, where the objective of the research was revealed fully to the respondents to gain spontaneous and self-revealing insight (Lazarsfeld, 1937; Rothwell, 1955).

2. **Projective techniques** mainly consisted of a word association test, a Thematic Appreciation Test and sentence completion test, and they were used in situations where it was likely for consumers to repress their feelings. Projective techniques involved presenting the respondents with an ambiguous stimulus and asking them to make sense of it, by doing what the respondents would need to fill in the gaps and project part of themselves into the stimulus, hence unknowingly revealed information about themselves (Haire, 1950).

The evolution of Motivation Research

Despite its inception in the 1930s, Motivation Research only took off in the early 1950s when it was legitimised by the American Marketing Association (Fullerton, 2013). It gained full support from the Marketing Research Techniques Committee in 1951 (Woodward et al., 1950), and was further legitimised by the Advertising Research Foundation in 1952, through a series of publications for advertising agencies. With extensive coverage and publications in the mainstream magazine *Business Week* in 1954, as well as the release of Vance Packard's highly controversial book, *The Hidden Persuaders*, in 1957, public attention to Motivation Research climaxed and it successfully gained extensive awareness amongst business managers (Fullerton, 2005).

By the mid-1950s, many large-scale organisations were already conducting Motivation Research to deep dive into the consumer psyche. The most prominent motivation researchers included many respected social scientists, such as S. B. Britt, B. B. Gardner, H. Herzog, P. Martineau, D. W. Twedt, W. L. Warner and L. Cheskin (Fullerton, 2013). These motivation researchers could be divided into three basic schools of thought, including Ernest Dichter, from the Freudian school, Warner from the more psychosocial perspective, and Herzog from a more female-inclusive perspective (Samuel, 2010).

Despite its popularity, Motivation Research remained controversial. In 1950, the Market Research Committee of the American Marketing Association alerted the marketing industry to the fact that some Motivation researchers had made un-substantiated claims and therefore critical assessments of their findings would be required. There was also concern as to the ability and willingness of academic social scientists to cooperate with business executives. Finally, the effectiveness, validity and reliability of the two most frequently employed Motivation Research methodologies, depth interview and projective techniques, were also being chal-lenged (Fullerton, 2013).

To add fuel to the fire, in his book, Vance Packard challenged the morality of Motivation Research as it enabled marketers to exploit consumers' weaknesses and manipulate them into irrational behaviours by invading into their unconscious thoughts without permission. Worst of all, Motivation Research also attempted to shape the character of the average American and encourage him in the direction of hedonism and self-indulgent materialism (Packard, 1957).

From the 1960s onwards, there was considerably less media attention given to Motivation Research and it became further de-emphasised as new methods for re-searching consumer behaviours appeared in the United States. With the advent of computer technology, the academic research field began to adopt more quantitative approaches. For example, sophisticated mathematical modelling, simulation and large-scale multivariate statistical analysis allowed researchers to analyse research results with greater power; besides, newer qualitative research, which made use of cultural anthropology in order to develop better questioning techniques also emerged (Fullerton, 2013). In addition, the development of MRI technology al-lowed a new neuromarketing field to emerge, which aimed to provide additional insights into the cognitive processing that affects consumer attitudes and behav-iours (Nelson, 2007).

Having said that, Motivation Research did not entirely disappear in the mar-keting and advertising industry. In fact, it has been continually reinvented and transformed into various different contemporary research methodologies, such as focus group discussions, lifestyle studies, anthropologic and ethnographic research (Horowitz, 1986; Schwarzkopf & Gries, 2010).

Ernest Dichter – the father of Motivation Research

Ernest Dichter was an Austrian psychologist born in Vienna in 1907. He studied psychoanalysis at the University of Vienna and obtained a doctorate in psychol-ogy in 1934. After studying and working with two practising psychoanalysts, Wilhelm Steckel and August Aichhorn, Dichter operated his own private psycho-analytic practice between 1934–1937 at Berggasse 20, across the street from where Freud lived, although Dichter never met Freud in person (Horowitz, 1986; Full-erton, 2013). Dichter emigrated to the United States in 1937. In 1939, he set up a consulting practice that specialised in finding the motivation triggers for consumer purchases, and he named his method 'Motivation Research' (Stern, 2004). In 1946, Dichter founded the Institute for Motivation Research in Croton-on-Hudson, New York and expanded throughout Switzerland and Germany in subsequent years. Dichter was generally recognised as the 'father' of Motivation Research due to high public profile and media exposure, even though he was not the true founder of Motivation Research. He pioneered the application of Freudian psychoanalysis to uncover consumers' hidden motivations, making his unique version of Motivation Research a powerful approach that allegedly could tap into the consumers' 'unconscious', to unearth their feelings about brands and products (Williams, 1957).

According to Dichter, true research must be interpretive in nature, and it must attempt to identify the true reason behind an attitude or a behaviour. However, many attitudes could not be verbalised easily, marketers must, therefore, use Motivation Research techniques to go beyond 'language-inhibited' statements to uncover the truth (Bartos, 1977). Dichter exchanged the classic 'four Ps' of marketing – product, price, place and promotion – with four Ss – sustenance, sex, security and status – claiming that these were the universal human drives determining all consumer behaviours. Dichter was an advocate of the 'pleasure principle' and hedonism and he argued that by freeing the id from rational reasoning, consumers could be rid of their deeply engrained puritanical ethics and obtain the necessary moral permission to enjoy the good things in life (Dichter, 1960). Dichter also asserted that all ordinary everyday goods had a psychic content and were loaded with symbolic meanings grounded in social and cultural significance. Therefore, to Dichter, wood was more than a material, as it signified life, glass symbolised uncertainty, ambiguity and mystery, shoes represented strength and independence, hair connoted potency and virility, thus, all products and brands were extensions of the consumers' personality (Samuel, 2010).

Dichter's view on why people smoked

In *The Psychology of Everyday Living*, Dichter (1947) devoted an entire chapter on why people smoked, although the entire book was later rejected by the psychoanalytic circle and regarded as of no value to the psychoanalysts, the clinical psychiatrist, or the general practitioner despite its wide circulation (Keiser, 1948). The following is a summary of Dichter's view on smoking and cigarettes.

Through hundreds of direct observations, depth interviews and projective tests, Dichter concluded that taste and quality were not the reason why smokers continued to smoke: it was the psychological pleasure and satisfaction smokers obtained from their cigarettes that mattered. According to Dichter, the act of smoking was heavily imbued with childhood wishes, symbolic meanings, and fundamental human needs. For example, smoking was fun because it served as a substitute for the childhood habit of following momentary impulses regardless of consequences – it was a legitimate excuse for interrupting work in order to steal a moment of pleasure. Smoking was also an oral pleasure and there was a direct connection between thumb-sucking and smoking – the satisfied expression on a smoker's face when they inhaled their cigarette was proof of a sensuous thrill derived from the oral pleasure of smoking.

A cigarette was also a reward that smokers could give themselves any time they wanted. The first and last cigarette of the day had significant symbolic meanings to smokers; the first cigarette represented a consolation prize in preparation for the hectic day ahead, and an excuse to postpone the start of the working day; the last cigarette of the day signified the moment where the door could be closed, and the smoker could finally rest and safely retreat to sleep. To many smokers, a cigarette was also used psychologically as a modern hourglass; the burning down of a cigarette resembled the marking of time and it also made time pass more quickly in situations where smokers were forced to be patient. In that sense, cigarettes might even have a psychotherapeutic effect in calming smokers down. Many smokers claimed that smoking helped them think and this perception could be explained by the fact that smoking provided a personal smokescreen, which helped to shut out distractions so that the mind could best concentrate. At the same time, smoking could also help smokers relax, because it was perceived as rhythmic, like music, and it gave them a legitimate excuse to linger a little longer after meals and to avoid working for a little longer. Furthermore, the act of deep inhalation and exhalation in smoking also helped relieve tension and low mood by forcing a rhythmic expansion of the chest, thus providing a calming function, and restoring the normal pace of breathing. This explained why some smokers believed that cigarettes helped provide relief and they could somehow 'blow their troubles away' with cigarettes.

Some of the appeal of lit cigarettes came from the smoke and the fire. Due to its fluidity, the smoke itself was charged with symbolic meanings related to mystery and magic. Many smokers expressed that they enjoyed watching the smoke they puffed out when smoking cigarettes; to them, the exhaled smoke seemed to represent a part of themselves. The act of smoking represented a co-creation process between the smokers and the cigarettes; the smoke was produced by the smokers, so it satisfied the human's innate and deep-rooted desire for creativity. Fire was regarded as the symbol of life and it was surrounded by much superstition. In modern times, it was considered bad luck to light three cigarettes with one match, because the story was told that in the First World War, three soldiers were lighting their cigarettes and the third soldier was hit when the match flared up for the last time.

Cigarettes also seemed to have a life of their own and appeared to be awakened when lit, so smoking cigarettes was like being with a friend, and one would never feel lonely with a cigarette. In our everyday lives, cigarettes also help break down social barriers and facilitate social conversation; besides, the custom of lighting another smoker's cigarette has also contained an erotic significance.

In the chapter, 'Why do we smoke cigarettes?' Dichter (1947) concluded that despite general agreement on the health risks associated with smoking, the psychological pleasure derived from smoking proved to be much more powerful than any religious, moral, and legal reasoning, and that a 'pleasure miracle' had so much to offer that one could safely predict that cigarettes were here to stay.

A critical evaluation of Motivation Research: theoretical, methodological, technical and ethical debates

From a theoretical perspective, with his overt emphasis on using sexual motivations to provide superficial interpretations and a generalisation of consumer behaviours based on limited evidence, Dichter violated one of the key scientific theories of psychoanalysis laid down by Freud. In 'wild' psychoanalysis (Freud, 1910), Freud reaffirmed that in psychoanalysis, the word 'sexuality' did not equate with genital orgasm and it was used to denote 'to love', similar to its meaning and usage in German. The expression 'sexual life' had a much wider meaning, including,

> ... all the activities of the tender feelings which have primitive sexual impulses as their source, even when those impulses have become inhibited in regard to their original sexual aim or have exchanged this aim for another which is no longer sexual. For this reason we prefer to speak of psychosexuality, thus laying stress on the point that the mental factor in sexual life should not be overlooked or underestimated.
>
> (Freud, 1910, pp. 222–223)

Freud went on to suggest that 'anyone not sharing this view of psychosexuality has no right to adduce psycho-analytic theses dealing with the aetiological importance of sexuality'.

From a methodological perspective, despite the popularity and influence of Motivation Research, it was built on three questionable assumptions: first, social sciences such as sociology and psychoanalysis possessed a body of research readily applicable to advertising and marketing; second, researchers in the commercial field had the skills to apply the methods; and third, the results could be generalised to the population. According to Winick (1955), these assumptions were flawed: in the first place, the number of proven laws in social science was small and most of them were undergoing continuous revision; taking projective tests as an example, even in a clinical setting where the patients had a strong motivation to help, the validity was only 30 per cent; second, years of training were required to produce a competent social interviewer, but most of the interviewers used in Motivation Research were either unemployed or recent graduate students who had no training or work experience. Finally, when different organisations commissioned Motivation Research on similar projects to different research companies, they usually received completely different, sometimes opposite, recommendations from different research companies, hence the results of Motivation Research were highly subjective and its generalisability questionable.

Winick's criticisms on Motivation Research were further reinforced by Rothwell (1955), who listed seven objections to the Motivation Researchers. These included the Motivation Researchers' attempts to advocate research for personal financial gain; a tendency to present conclusions based on a partially confirmed hunch with no intention of providing validation; failure to present any supporting evidence of their findings and recommendations; an unwillingness to acknowledge other drivers in economic, anthropological, and statistical disciplines and only a rigid focus on psychology; the inclination to present Motivation Research as a silver bullet for all marketing issues, disregarding all other types of research; their propensity to conceal a limited sample size; and finally, their tendency to distort and dramatise the results of their recommendations for business, which could well be a manifestation of the Hawthorne effect (Sonnenfeld, 1985), whereby an increase in sales could be totally unrelated to the recommendations made by the Motivation Researchers.

From a technical perspective, the over-reliance on projective techniques and depth interviews in deriving marketing recommendations in Motivation Research also attracted many criticisms from the research field. To be specific, even in a clinical setting where trained clinical psychologists were aided by a wealth of personal background information about their patients, it was always difficult for them to differentiate projective test results upon which their patients would really act, between those which merely served as a substitute for action. In a market research context, this meant the 'unconscious' drives to purchase a product revealed in projective tests might not lead to real purchase action (Lindzey, 1952). Furthermore, other problems associated with projective tests included first, that the produced results were heavily affected by momentary environmental and personal factors of the interviewers and respondents, by the interaction between them, by time and place of tests, and by what methods the results were analysed. To what extent these momentary impulses would last long enough to result in an intention or actual action to purchase a product was therefore questionable. Moreover, there was a lack of normative data for all projective tests except the Rorschach test, which in turn undermined the objective appraisal of the information obtained. Finally, it was debatable whether the interviewers and analysts of commercial market research firms were qualified to conduct proper projective tests, as this issue was further complicated by the fact that the proper administration of projective tests required an unhurried and relaxed atmosphere, and a large number of carefully selected and standardised pictures was required to identify a consistent pattern, which was something that the commercial interviews and analysts lacked (Rothwell, 1955).

Depth interviews, another key technique employed by the Motivation Researchers, could also suffer from serious distortion in interpretation. The risk was intensified with the lack of an evaluation methodology to justify the results yielded by Motivation Research, and what marketers and advertisers obtained from Motivation Researchers could be just the result of a hunch rather than actual insight, based on the 'unconscious' drivers of consumers (Rothwell, 1955). An underlying assumption of depth interviews was that the 'unconscious' could be tapped into in these short sessions, leading to the identification of hidden motives. However, it must be noted that there was a huge difference between the psychoanalytic session and the depth interview session, so the 'unconscious' suggested by Freud could not possibly be the 'unconscious' alluded to by Motivation Research. The main difference is in the motivation context that led to a conversation between two people in these sessions. In the psychoanalytic treatment, the patient consults the psychoanalyst in order to resolve the acute pain resulting from their neurotic disorder. The aim of the treatment is to allow for re-admission of the repressed elements into the patient's consciousness. This process is extremely painful, and takes years of treatment for the patient to accept the painful reality as a lesser evil than neurotic pain. On the contrary, the motivation context in depth interview consultation was reversed, that is, the consumer does not seek help, instead the interviewer looks to the consumer and has a business motive. As such, the consumer who attends a depth interview has much less need to open up than the patient in a psychoanalytic session, thus, it was highly questionable whether the 'unconscious' could be revealed in such a low-intensity context. In addition, as the 'unconscious' that Freud referred to took years to unearth, it was highly debatable that an interview session of a few short hours, it would be able to reveal such material (Politz, 1956).

Despite the theoretical, methodological, technical, and ethical debates, the ideas established by Motivation Research continue to be a significant influence on the practices of the advertising industry in the 21st century. First, Motivation researchers were the first to stress the importance of image and persuasion rather than product in advertising, and it is now commonly understood in the marketing and advertising industry that products are an extension of the character traits of consumers, and may therefore be seen as an expression of their personality; The Coca-Cola Company sells the idea of youth, refreshment and celebration rather than the product of carbonated soft drinks, and the Nike Corporation sells exertion, achievement and success rather than simply pairs of sneakers. Second, Motivation Research continues to be used by research practitioners (Levy 2003, 2005), and it is regarded as a pre-cursor to various contemporary research methodologies, such as focus group research, lifestyle studies, and anthropologic and ethnographic research (Horowitz, 1986; Tadajewski, 2006; Schwarzkopf & Gries, 2010). Finally, Motivation Research has laid the foundations of the study of consumer behaviour as a discipline today (Fullerton, 2013). J. F. Engel, who published an article called 'Motivation research – magic or menace?' on the merit of Motivation Research in 1961, later became the lead author on the pioneering textbook on consumer behaviour, in which the organisation of topics was taken directly from Motivation Research (Fullerton, 2013).

In spite of its general adoption in contemporary marketing, advertising and marketing research, and the fact that it did provide some interesting observations on smoking behaviours, such as the act of smoking being heavily imbued with childhood wishes, symbolic meanings, and fundamental human needs, and therefore, the taste and quality of the cigarettes were not the reason why smokers continued to smoke, Motivation Research did not explain the psychological origins of highly addictive behaviours. For example, why would a cigarette, rather than any other product, be chosen as an object to satisfy childhood wishes, and why is the act of smoking infused with so many symbolic meanings? Furthermore, with its over-reliance on sexual impulses and drives in accounting for consumer behaviours, Motivation Researchers neglected the vital role played by social factors in driving consumer behaviours in general and smoking addiction in particular. Therefore, Motivation Research findings do not appear to add much value to the understanding of our research question on smoking addiction.

Chapter 4

Psychoanalytic understanding

Let us now turn to the psychoanalytic understanding of smoking addiction. We will briefly cover the Freudian and Kleinian views on smoking addiction, followed by a review of the later psychoanalytic literature.

The Freudian view

Mummy, my smoking addiction is an oral fixation because you weaned me at the wrong time!

Sigmund Freud, the father of psychoanalysis, was well known for his helpless addiction to cigar smoking. The famous quote attributed to him, 'sometimes a cigar is just a cigar' (Marcovitz 1969, p. 1083), suggests how much Freud enjoyed smoking, to the extent that he was willing to deny all the symbolic meanings to the practice. In fact, cigar smoking is a running theme in Freud's diary, and he was unable to work unless he smoked a cigar (Larsen, 1997). Peter Gay's major biography of Freud, recounts that Freud once told his nephew Harry, aged 17, on declining a cigarette offered to him by his uncle, 'my boy, smoking is one of the greatest and cheapest enjoyments in life, and if you decide in advance not to smoke, I can only feel sorry for you' (Gay, 1988, p. 178). In 1923, at the age of 67, Freud was diagnosed with oral cancer and endured a total of 33 exhausting and painful operations in the remaining 16 years of his life (The oral cancer foundation, 2010). Despite numerous ultimatums issued by his doctor, Freud continued to smoke knowing that smoking would eventually kill him.

All forms of addiction, in Freud's view, are substitutes for masturbation, which is the 'primal addiction' imbued with sexual phantasies; smoking addiction is a result of infantile 'oral fixation' caused by premature or delayed weaning by the mother (Freud, 1897).

DOI: 10.4324/9781003329077-7

The Kleinian view

I introject (inhale) my cigarette to protect myself from the terrifying bad objects in my internal world.

Melanie Klein, who is called 'the mother of the Objects Relations Theory' in psychoanalysis, did not publish research on addiction; but Herbert Rosenfeld, a close collaborator of Klein, did draw on the Kleinian framework and postulated a Kleinian view on drug addiction.

Rosenfeld (1960) suggested that because the drug addict's ego is too weak to bear the pain of depression caused by loss of the good internal object – without it, his internal world is instead populated by terrifying, internal bad objects, goodness is outweighed by badness. Such depression is experienced unconsciously by the addict as an internal deadness and deep emptiness, as if a sense of being alive has been threatened, which can only be relieved by consuming things, this includes eating, bingeing, tobacco, and smoke, to protect the internal ego (Hinshelwood, 1991). This act of 'taking things in' in a concrete way enables the addict to hallucinate the calling-in of external reinforcements for protection against persecutory, internal bad objects. In this sense, cigarette can then be seen as, at least by smokers, as an external good object that can prevent the internal ego from disintegration and complete annihilation And of course, one can make the link between cancer and the internal deadness, which makes it such a potent anxiety that it must be denied as it is much too terrifying.

According to Rosenfeld, this regressed state is:

> … a phase of infancy where the infants use hallucinatory wish-fulfilment phantasies in dealing with their anxieties. This state is closely related to the manic mechanisms and defences, and the drug effect being used as an artificial physical aid in the production of the hallucination, in the same way as the infant uses its fingers or thumb as an aid to hallucinating the ideal breast.
>
> (Rosenfeld, 1960, p. 468)

Later psychoanalytic literature

There has been a considerable number of papers published in the psychoanalytic field on the psychodynamics behind addiction, and in particular drug addiction. A total of 78 hits have been identified through a PEP-Web search on 'addiction', which can be divided into four clusters: the first cluster of literature links addiction to an expression of the derivatives of the repressed drives including oral fixations, latent homosexuality, narcissistic factors, aggression, and paranoid characteristics; the second cluster views addiction as an ego function to compensate for the absence of a good internal object; the third cluster focuses on the exploration of addiction to various behaviours and mental states; the fourth cluster shows an attempt to re-conceptualise addiction from different theoretical paradigms.

Cluster 1: addiction as an expression of the derivatives of the repressed drives

- Radó (1926, 1928), Daniels (1933), Robbins (1935), and Benedek (1936) confirmed oral factors in addiction.
- Abraham (1926) and Riggall (1923) linked drug addiction and alcoholism to latent homosexuality.
- Abraham (1926) explored the psychological relations between sexuality and alcoholism.
- Radó (1933) reviewed the vicissitudes of the ego and placed emphasis on narcissistic factors in drug addiction.
- Menninger (1934) explored the psychoanalytic origin of surgical compulsion and linked it to a gratification of the patient's unconscious needs for surgical castrations.
- Abraham (1926), Glover (1932), and Simmel (1948) emphasised on aggressive factors and the early oedipal conflict in addiction.
- Freud (1917), Radó (1926), Benedek (1936), Simmel (1948), Glover (1932) and Crowley (1939) explored the paranoid aspect of addiction.

Cluster 2: addiction as compensation for a weak ego function

- Rosenfeld (1960) connected drug addiction to manic-depressive illness.
- Khantzian's (1987) 'self-medication hypothesis' suggested that addiction is a manifestation of an early failure to internalise self-care from parents, and due to the lack of these internalisations, addicts are unable to regulate and tolerate affects such as self-esteem or relationships and therefore they use drugs to self-medicate and compensate for their inability to tolerate affects.
- Other ego functions of drug addiction include using the drug as a substitute for a lost object or idealised object (Schur, 1963; Frosch, 1970); to compulsively re-create or deal with an early trauma or dangerous situation in a controllable environment in order to gain mastery over it (Szasz, 1958; Robinson & Berridge, 2003; Johnson, 2003); to serve as a method of self-punishment to ease the sense of oedipal guilt (Harris, 1964); to defend against the super-ego (De Paula Ramos, 2004); to serve as an external soothing agent (Fleming, 2005); to combat feelings of intolerable helplessness and disintegration (Savitt, 1963; Dodes, 1990, 2003; Johnson, 1999; Khantzian, 2005); to deal with failure in internalisation (Khantzian, 1978), and to re-establish a symbiotic fusion experience as a result of disturbed early object relationships and the fear of good internal objects being overpowered by bad ones (Woollcott, 1981).

- Zinberg (1975) investigated the impact of social settings on ego function and drug effect.

Cluster 3: addiction to various behaviours and mental states

- Addiction to alternative belief systems (Cath, 1982).
- Addiction to near death (Joseph, 1983; Gottdiener, 2006).
- Addiction to perfection (Woodman, 1982).
- Addiction to the love relationship (Haaken, 1992).
- Some explored the processes and casual relationships in addiction (Adler, 1986; Khantzian, 1987; Lane, et al., 1991; Hopper, 1995; Gabbard, 2002), and the relationship between creativity and addiction (Knafo, 2008).

Cluster 4: conceptualisation of addiction from different theoretical perspectives

- Ulman and Paul (2013) suggested that addiction is a manifestation of dependence on 'Addictive Trigger Mechanisms' to produce a dissociative and altered sense of self and to provide desperately needed antianxiety and antidepressant self-object functions'.
- Dodes (1996) viewed addiction as a subset of compulsion.
- Bornstein (1996) re-conceptualised addiction based on an integrated object relations/interactionist model of dependency.
- Jacobson (2003) regarded sexual addiction as a form of perversion.

Amongst the various forms of addiction, smoking is the most unique: there is the absence of a similar physical withdrawal syndrome that is usually associated with alcohol, sedative, opioid, and stimulant addiction upon smoking cessation, and there is no markedly increased consumption once smokers reach a certain consumption quantity. The above suggests that compared to other types of addiction, smoking addiction seems to be more heavily dependent on psychological factors rather than pharmacological factors.

Added to the intricacy of the dynamics of smoking addiction is that, because a cigarette is a legal consumer product with high turnover, unlike other addictive substances which are either strictly banned from any form of direct sale to consumers, or heavily regulated by the government; cigarette consumption has been widely advertised by the tobacco companies as a glamorous and aspirational symbol, and there is also a common belief that tobacco advertising plays a key role in promoting the persistence of smoking addiction.

Despite the rich psychoanalytic literature on addiction, very little has been written on smoking addiction in particular. Only nine papers have been identified by a PEP-Web search and most of these focused on confirming the oral origin of smoking and an obsession with masturbation, exploring the symbolic meaning of smoking, or linking it with the expression of a death wish and the depressive loss of internal life. None of the papers located attempted to investigate the aetiology of smoking addiction.

Symbolic meaning of smoking

- Brill (1922) supported Freud's view on the oral origin of smoking.
- Hiller (1922) provided various symbolic meanings of smoking and suggested that cigarettes, cigars and pipes represent a substitute for the penis or the breast that the smokers were deprived of in childhood, hence the smokers started to smoke because of the phallic significance of cigarettes which reminded them of their childhood deprivation.
- Green (1923), on the other hand, linked smoking to the expression of a death wish.
- Berent (1961) emphasised the ritualistic aspect and the forepleasure of smoking.
- Marcovitz (1969) postulated that heavy cigarette smoking is a respiratory addiction, rather than an oral addiction comprising the respiratory triad of inhalation – exhalation – visualisation, which was supported by a subsequent comparative study (Grotjahn, 1972).

Chapter 5

Psychoanalytically informed cross-disciplinary perspectives

In spite of the limited number of papers written directly about smoking addiction and listed on PEP-Web, if we turn to the marketing and social science field as a basis for a literature search, there is evidence of an early influence from the field of psychoanalysis on the understanding of smoking addiction. Such works include the 'torch of freedom' public relations campaign developed by Edward Bernays in the 1920s. Bernays was Freud's nephew and is often called 'the father of Public Relations'. A landmark ice cream study in the 1950s by Isabel Menzies Lyth explored psychoanalytic meaning behind the consumption of 'pleasure food', that is, ice cream and tobacco, from the perspective of the Object Relations School.

Edward Bernays' view

A cigarette is the 'torch of freedom' for the modern liberated women

The application of psychoanalytic concepts in the marketing and advertising field started in the 1920s when Edward Bernays constructed the theoretical foundation of modern public relations – an important tool in the marketing mix. In his pioneering book *Propaganda*, Bernays (1928, p. 37) stated:

> The conscious and intelligent manipulation of the organized habits and opinions of the masses is an important element in democratic society. Those who manipulate this unseen mechanism of society constitutes an invisible government which is the true ruling power of our country.

Bernays made it very clear that the objective of public relations is to manipulate public opinion in order to achieve a certain objective, and those '… who understand the mental processes and social patterns of the masses. It is they who pull the wires that control the public mind' (Bernays, 1928, p. 38). As the nephew of Freud, it was widely known that Bernays actively made use of Freud's theories of psychoanalysis, especially the impact of the unconscious in forming his public relations strategy.

DOI: 10.4324/9781003329077-8

In the 1920s, Bernays was hired by the American Tobacco Company, one of the original mother companies forming today's British American Tobacco Company, in order to develop a public relations campaign promoting cigarette consumption amongst women. After consulting the psychoanalyst A. A. Brill (Torches of Freedom Campaign, n.d), Bernays leveraged the unconscious desire of women to be liberated from their stereotypical roles and launched the legendary 'Torches of Freedom' public relations campaign. He hired a group of beautiful female fashion models to march in the New York City parade, each waving a lit Lucky Strike cigarette and wearing a banner declaring their cigarettes to be a 'torch of freedom'. The campaign achieved unprecedented media coverage and helped break the social taboo of women smoking in public, establishing the cigarette as a symbol of liberation.

Bernays' insight into the power of marketing and advertising in the manipulation of the unconscious provided a good starting point in understanding how people may be led away from conscious attitudes and thoughts. This makes psychoanalysis a means to understand the unconscious and provide possible explanations of the apparent irrationality of smoking addiction, although Bernays himself did not publish any related study on smoking addiction.

Isabel Menzies Lyth's view

The cigarette is a miracle 'pleasure food' that has the power to transform anxiety into pleasure.

The 1950s marked the beginning of the psychoanalytic contribution to marketing and advertising from the British Object Relations School, which provided new levers to the understanding of consumption and smoking addiction. To be specific, the psychoanalytic framework shifted from emphasis on sexual pleasures derived from the satisfaction of instinctual drive to pre-genital sucking pleasures derived from relating to objects, as evident in the contributions of Menzies Lyth detailed in the next section

Between 1950 and 1970, the Tavistock Institute of Human Relations (TIHR), a sister institution to the Tavistock Clinic, was approached by many major companies for the development and marketing of their products, which marked the beginning of TIHR's explorations, from a British Object Relations perspective, as to what motivated consumers to buy things. From then onwards, a diversity of pioneering studies on consumer behaviours utilising Object Relations' psychoanalytic ideas emerged. Amongst the many research projects undertaken by the TIHR, the study on the associative links between ice cream, milk, and the breast by Menzies Lyth using a Kleinian Object Relations approach seems to bear the highest relevance on the understanding of smoking addiction, since both ice cream and cigarettes can be grouped under a special category of food called 'pleasure foods.'

In *Envy and gratitude and other works 1946–1963*, Klein (1975, p. 95) stated that 'the infant's relations to his first object, the mother, and towards food are bound up with each other from the beginning'. This view was taken up and further developed by Menzies Lyth in a landmark ice cream study commissioned by an advertising agency and their client in 1950 to discover how to increase sales of ice cream during the winter. Using the technique of group discussions derived by Bion and pioneered at TIHR (Miller & Rose, 1997), a random group of potential consumers were recruited for a discussion on their consumption of ice cream. The sessions were facilitated by a moderator and the verbatim accounts were transcribed by another researcher in the room. With this technique, a kind of free association by the consumers emerged, starting with practical questions and later veering off into the underlying unconscious dynamics of ice cream consumption, which involved many more complex forces than the ice cream manufacturer had originally envisaged, rendering their intention to increase winter sales via penetration of the family meal system at home, an extremely difficult task.

As reported in Menzies Lyth and Trist's 'The development of ice cream as a food' (Menzies Lyth & Trist, 1989), ice cream could be consumed either at home or on external premises. For home consumption, it was revealed in the group that only three per cent of homes had refrigerators, and none had home freezers, which made the idea of home consumption of ice cream an unrealistic target. Some respondents even complained about the teasing quality of ice cream advertisements, which encouraged home consumption. In addition, there were also problems for the inclusion of ice cream in the family meal system. For housewives, providing ice cream as a dessert in the family meal triggered a sense of guilt, because ice cream was an off-the-shelf, ready-to-eat item, so housewives did not need to do anything to prepare it. Therefore, serving ice cream was seen as an attack on their role as the provider of food in the family, and hence in conflict with their wish to sustain that feeding role. Furthermore, ice cream was seen as a competitor to custard, a foodstuff that housewives made themselves, and serving ice cream involved a visible additional cost, hence an additional financial burden to the family, whereas custard cost nothing in the eyes of the housewives, because it was made from 'free' ingredients already available at home.

Menzies Lyth (1989) also referred to Melanie Klein's work on the 'internal world' and argued that the 'internal society' was the bridge between the psychological and the social, as an external stimulus had to be taken in and experienced inside in order for it to exert any significant influence on the individual. The notion of the 'internal society' had a substantial impact on behaviours related to food and eating, because the experience of feeding and one's emotional relationship with the mother were intimately linked, and these early experiences also formed the major components of the 'internal society'. Therefore, eating was not purely an isolated act to obtain nourishment, it should also be regarded as a major social and emotional activity for all human beings, because people always eat in the context of the 'internal society'.

In the same paper, Menzies Lyth put forward the concept of 'pleasure foods', which was a synthesis between Kurt Lewin's field theory, that is, the impact of environmental factors, and psychoanalysis, namely, the internal environment through which the consumers responded to field forces. According to Menzies Lyth:

Ice cream belongs to a group of products which may be described as pleasure foods. Other products in this group are chocolates and sweets, alcoholic and soft

drinks, and many kinds of preserves, sweetmeats and desserts. Closely associated, though not actually eaten or drunk, are tobacco and chewing gum. These
products are related to certain psychological and social factors and characteristic of them is their ability to gratify oral desires and, like the breast with the
infant, change depression and anxiety into pleasure.

(Menzies Lyth, 1989, pp. 71–72)

To Menzies Lyth, ice cream was 'the pleasure food par excellence' because of its
symbolic resemblance to the breast and the mother-infant relationship. The consumption of pleasure food involves

a situation where the realistic nutritional use of food may be submerged by its
use to increase pleasure and reduce pain within relationships. Food is used to
mediate and to symbolise relationships ... food is a relationship substitute ... the
ritual of the bedtime drink is often linked with the longing for a good internal
mother-baby relationship through the emphasis on milk, on the feeding proper-
ties of the drink and on its sweetness. The drink establishes the symbol of a good
mother inside who will give or protect the good experiences of sleep or even life
itself, since many people seem to fear that sleep will deepen into death.

(Menzies Lyth, 1989, pp. 62–64)

Menzies Lyth pointed out that commercial advertising is usually able to leverage these widespread social patterns in a sophisticated, sensitive, and impactful
manner that reinforces these deep-rooted patterns with commercial success. One
classic example (1956) of how advertising cleverly exploited how we dealt with
our relationship gap can be seen in the advertising campaign, 'Bridge that gap with
a Cadbury's snack'. Even though the gap appears to be a hunger gap, the latent
unconscious gap is in fact a relationship gap, and by eating a snack one can temporarily bridge the gap between our internal and external societies using food, which
matches how people usually deal with separations in their internal and external
societies.

In early mother-infant interactions, the infant learned to establish primitive casual relationships between food, feeding, the mother, and emotional experiences;
taking in good food from a good mother aroused positive emotional experiences
and alleviated bad ones; lacking food from a bad mother evoked negative emotional experiences and reduced good ones. These primitive causal connections continued to exert their influences as the infant grew up, even though the memories
remained unconscious. Oral gratification through the consumption of 'pleasure
foods' triggered both conscious and unconscious memories of the early feeding relationship with the mother, which in turn helped to reduce anxieties and depression
derived from the primitive infantile anxiety and depression associated with the loss
of the good object, that is, the breast. Hence, the consumption of 'pleasure foods'
was regarded as a compensation for the loss of the breast, and its need was most
acute in situations that awakened these primitive needs. The food value of these
'pleasure foods' was only secondary in comparison to the psychological pleasure

they provided through the oral gratification related to early psychological experiences. This group of 'pleasure foods' included chocolates and sweets, alcoholic and carbonated soft drinks, preserves, sweetmeats and desserts, as well as tobacco and chewing gum, even though they were not physically swallowed.

Due to strong connections between food, interpersonal relationships, and emotional experiences, food was sometimes used as a relationship substitute to deal with separation anxieties aroused in external and internal societies, resulting in detachment from its nutritional value:

> This kind of oral gratification serves then as a method of alleviating current anxieties and depression which are in part the derivatives of the infantile anxiety and depression connected with the actual loss of the breast. Compensation for this loss is sought in the consumption of substitute objects, the pleasure foods. Thus, the need for them becomes particularly great when contemporary difficulties awaken again the residues of the earlier situations which to a greater or lesser extent exist in anyone.
>
> (Menzies Lyth, 1989, p. 72)

Thus, pleasure foods are used to increase pleasure and reduce pain in an interpersonal relationship, instead of being consumed for nutritional value. The danger of such detachment was manifold. First, it disturbed the control systems that regulated nutritional signals and nutritional needs, resulting in obesity or malnutrition or both. Second, the foods that satisfied emotional instead of nutritional needs usually contained high carbohydrates and refined sugar, which caused a rapid elevation of blood sugar, hence creating the experience of immediate physical and emotional uplift. Due to the very nature of these 'pleasure foods', people could easily become addicted to them without being aware of it. Psychoanalytic explanations of such an addiction could be that in their attempt to deny the depriving and frustrating internal mother linked with the carbohydrates, the addict wanted to prove that their mother was capable of giving food, therefore they forced her to give what she could not or would not give, which could lead to disastrous results. In postscript of the same paper, Menzies Lyth explained how addiction in the consumption of pleasure food including tobacco could lead to dangerous outcomes.

> When this paper was originally written, pleasure foods, with the possible exception of alcohol, could be regarded as a relatively innocent way to relieve anxiety and distress, with good nutrition as a bonus. Unfortunately, this is no longer the case; so many of the ingredients of the pleasure foods are now suspect: sugar, animal fats, chocolate; tobacco can actually be a killer, and alcohol can be dangerous except in small amounts.
>
> (Menzies Lyth, 1989, pp. 87–88)

Given the psychoanalytically charged emotions behind the consumption of ice cream, Menzies Lyth pointed out that 'pleasure food' was 'intensely connected with primitive pleasure situations at the breast' and it has a 'great power to act as a substitute for the breast, to wipe out anxieties and depression' (Menzies Lyth 1989, p. 73). Hence, consumer consumption behaviours are characterised as the overwhelming need to combine all the pleasure foods to achieve the greatest pleasure in one go, like the primitive infantile greed, and the need to reassure oneself by having all the good things exclusively for oneself. There are a few points to note in the consumption experience of this special kind of 'pleasure food'. Specifically, ice cream could not be served too cold, for it would turn pleasure into a neuralgic pain, and the good object into a bad one, resulting in hatred and attack. Besides, because of consumers' infantile concrete thinking and the lack of the concept of object permanence, the absence of immediate availability of ice cream to satisfy the consumers' impulsive desire would likely trigger violent infantile hostility against the ice cream manufacturer, as such easy availability, that is, the magic appearance of the breast on desire, was more important than good taste which implied quality.

Part III

What does smoking addiction have to do with Linus's security blanket?

Amongst all the psychoanalytic theorists, D. W. Winnicott has provided a unique view by pointing out that 'addiction can be stated in terms of regression to the early stage at which the transitional phenomena are unchallenged' (Winnicott, 1953, p. 97).

In this part, we will provide a brief overview of Winnicott's biographical background, his key contributions to psychoanalytic theories and clinical practices, as well as a critical evaluation of his work, especially with respect to the transitional object and transitional phenomena which are closely linked to addiction in Winnicott's theoretical framework.

Key sections

- D. W. Winnicott: who was he?
- What are D. W. Winnicott's major contributions to psychoanalysis?
- What is D. W. Winnicott's view on smoking addiction?

DOI: 10.4324/9781003329077-9

Chapter 6

D. W. Winnicott

Who was he?

On the main landing page of PEP-Web, D. W. Winnicott's three landmark papers 'Transitional Objects and Transitional Phenomena – A Study of the First Not-Me Possession' (1953), 'Hate in the Counter-Transference' (1949) and 'The Theory of the Parent-Infant Relationship' (1960) are consistently ranked as the top three most searched papers, ahead of Melanie Klein's 'Notes on Some Schizoid Mechanisms' (1946), indicating his widespread popularity in the academic and research field.

Donald Winnicott was born on 7 April 1896 in Plymouth, Devon, into a prosperous family. He was the youngest child of three, having two older sisters. In 1923, at the age of 27, Winnicott joined the Paddington Green Children's Hospital and Queen Elizabeth Hospital, Hackney, starting his career as a child physician and staying there for 40 years. He also opened a private practice so he could see the patients he was particularly interested in. Winnicott spent most of his time working in these three clinics, and by the time he retired, he had worked with over 60,000 cases (Jacobs, 1995).

In 1934, Winnicott qualified as an adult psychoanalyst at the British Psychoanalytical Society, and as a child psychoanalyst the following year. He was the society's only male child analyst as well as a paediatrician at that time (Paskauskas, 1993). Winnicott had an initial association with Klein and was her student for five years; he was named by Klein as one of the five Kleinian training analysts during the period of the 'controversial discussions' between 1942 and 1944. During the same period, Winnicott became a psychiatric consultant for the Government Evacuation Scheme in Oxfordshire and this experience further inspired Winnicott to include the impact of the environment upon his own theoretical psychoanalytic framework (Davis & Wallbridge, 1981). During his lifetime, Winnicott was able to reach a wide audience, especially with his series of radio broadcast talks for the BBC at various times during the Second World War and the later 1940s.

Winnicott was a highly creative and original thinker. His ideas on the transitional object and transitional phenomena have attracted pervasive interests inside and outside the academic field, and his squiggle game procedure represented a ground-breaking approach for clinicians in therapeutic work with children. During his lifetime, he made a significant shift in Freud's concept of illusion, turning it into

DOI: 10.4324/9781003329077-10

a positive indicator, and he also adapted Klein's play therapy to include the spatula game with infants and mothers in clinical settings.

Despite these original contributions to the psychoanalytic field, Winnicott did not see himself as being original, and he was never interested in precedence. In *Collected papers: through paediatrics to psychoanalysis*, Winnicott says that:

> I shall not first give a historical survey and show the development of my ideas from the theories of others, because my mind does not work that way. What happens is that I gather this and that, here and there, settle down to clinical experience, form my own theories, and then, last of all, interest myself to see where I stole what.
>
> (Winnicott, 1975, p. 145)

In *The maturational process and the facilitating environment: studies in the theory of emotional development*, he writes:

> First I wish to acknowledge my debt to my psychoanalytic colleagues. I have grown up as a member of this group, and after so many years of inter-relating it is now impossible for me to know what I have learned and what I have contributed. The writings of any one of us must be to some extent plagiaristic. Nevertheless I think we do not copy; we work and observe and think and discover, even if it can be shown that what we discover has been discovered before.
>
> (Winnicott, 1965b, p. 11)

To another correspondent, he writes:

> I sometimes come around to feel compelled to work in my own way and to express myself in my own language first; by a struggle I sometimes come round to reworking what I am saying to bring it in line with other work, in which case I usually find that my own 'original' ideas were not so original as I had to think when they were emerging.
>
> (Rodman, 1987, pp. 53–54).

Even though Winnicott did not refer much to others' ideas in his papers, he was aware of the influence that other theorists had on him and did not lay claim to complete originality. As observed by Jacobs (1995), Winnicott's thinking was influenced by Darwin, Freud, and Klein, in chronological order, but he always transformed their theories with a perspective that was uniquely his own.

Inspired by Darwin's natural adaptation and selection process in evolutionary theory, Winnicott sees the mother (the environment of the baby) as continuously adapting to the needs of the baby, by gradually introducing the world in small doses to it, facilitating its progression from absolute dependence to relative dependence. For Winnicott, human development is a struggle against compliance with the environment, and this is the part where Winnicott reverses the Darwin equation (Phillips, 1988).

Despite his admiration for Freud, Winnicott moves away from Freud's father-child relationship to the mother-infant nursing couple, from the centrality of the Oedipus complex to the early mother-infant relationship, from an over-emphasis on drive and instinct and phantasy to the centrality of needs and environmental provision. He also replaces the psychosexual developmental stages of childhood with an emphasis on the tasks involved in ego development towards maturity and independence.

Winnicott was a student of Melanie Klein and under her supervision for six years from 1935–1941 (Jacobs, 2008). In *The maturational process and the facilitating environment: studies in the theory of emotional development* (1965b) he details Klein's key contributions to psychoanalysis, including the use of toys and play to understand the child's inner world, introjections and projections, inner and outer worlds, the persecutory internal objects, primitive defences, the capacity for concern, and the reparative outcome of guilt. Notwithstanding the above appreciations, Winnicott rejects the death instinct and opposes an emphasis on constitutional factors and phantasy.

Chapter 7

What are D. W. Winnicott's major contributions to psychoanalysis?

D. W. Winnicott was a prolific writer of short papers and he kept detailed case notes. He was not, however so much an author of extensively developed books, and unlike Freud and Klein, there is a lack of defined structure in his psychoanalytic theory. Having said that, one can still detect a sequence and distil major areas from the published work. Based on his 1965 book, *The maturational processes and the facilitating environment: studies in the theory of emotional development*, his ideas can be summarised under three main areas including: the developmental journey towards maturity, the task of mothering, and things that can go wrong during the developmental process, which we shall describe in detail in the following chapter.

Key sections

- The developmental journey towards maturity
- The task of mothering
- What can go wrong in the developmental process?

The developmental journey towards maturity

Psyche-soma indwelling

Winnicott asserts that in every child, there is an innate growth towards health and maturity, provided that there is a 'good enough' environment to contain and facilitate the development. To begin with, there needs to be a body-mind unity, and a process of 'dwelling of the psyche in the body' (Winnicott, 1988b, p. 123), an essential achievement many people would take for granted. In the infant, the psyche gradually comes to terms with the body through accumulations of personal experiences, such as physical impulses, sensations of the skin and muscular exercise, as well as environmental experiences, including how the mother holds the baby securely in order to allow sufficient time for it to adjust to gravity, something which is very new and alien to the baby. Generally speaking, a normal infant is firmly rooted

DOI: 10.4324/9781003329077-11

in the body only occasionally, even at one year old, for the psyche of the infant may easily lose touch with its body when, for example, it wakes up from deep sleep. It can explain for example, why mothers gradually wake up the infant before lifting it up to alleviate the unspeakable panic that can come upon waking, when the psyche has not caught up with the new position of the body (Winnicott, 1965a). Therefore, body-mind unity at the beginning of life cannot be taken for granted and the progression towards this stage of unity is a major developmental milestone.

Ego integration

Winnicott did not follow Freud's tripartite structural model of the psyche that regards the theoretical constructs of the id, ego and super-ego psychic apparatus, developed at different stages in our lives, whose interactions and activities govern our mental life. Winnicott openly contradicted Freud's model writing that, 'there is no id before ego' (1965b, p. 56). To Winnicott, the infant is unintegrated at the very beginning, it is without a definitive conscious and unconscious, and all the infant has is 'an armful of anatomy and physiology, and added to this a potential for development into a human personality' (Winnicott, 1988a, p. 89). Therefore, the ego does not exist at the beginning, its development depends on good-enough mothering to provide sufficient support for the early ego, in order to hold the infant and contain its unthinkable anxieties including:

1. going to pieces,
2. falling forever,
3. having no relationship to the body,
4. having no orientation, and
5. complete isolation because there is no means of communication.

(Winnicott, 1965b, p. 58; 1988a, pp. 98–99)

Ego integration relies on good-enough holding of the mother, allowing for a development of a sense of time and space, linking the baby with the physical body and the bodily functions, organising these sensory motor events into an internal psychic reality, and finding good objects, such as the breast and milk in the environment. When ego integration is combined with the feeling of body-mind unity and the psyche is able to dwell within the body sufficiently, then a 'satisfactory personalisation' is achieved (Winnicott, 1975, p. 151).

As the baby achieves a stronger body-mind unity over time, a growing sense of 'I am' emerges, which leads to a recognition of 'me/not me'. Becoming 'I am' and recognising the 'not me' as external is a developmental achievement, and 'only those who have reached a stage at which they can make this assertion are really qualified as adult members of society' (Winnicott, 1986, p. 141), although 'it will be understood that in practice these things develop gradually, and repeatedly come and go, and are achieved and lost' (Winnicott, 1965b, p. 216).

Absolute dependence to relative dependence, towards independence

Winnicott's description of personality development has no explicit links to Freud's threefold psychosexual stages of oral, anal, and phallic, nor to Klein's paranoid-schizoid and depressive positions. Winnicott's emphasis is on dependence and independence, and his scheme consists of three progressive categories, including absolute dependence, relative dependence and 'towards independence' (Winnicott, 1965b, p. 84). These three stages are progressive and continuous in nature, and any impingement during the developmental process is destined to lead to problems in the future.

Absolute dependence is a stage where 'there is no such thing as a baby' (Winnicott, 1964, p. 88). What can be seen is always a nursing couple, because a baby cannot exist alone without its mother, who is in a state of 'primary maternal occupation' (Winnicott, 1964, p. 300) in order to match with the baby's absolute dependence. The baby has a sense of omnipotence at this stage, believing that it has created everything it wants, so the mother's role is to assist the baby in creating the illusion of omnipotence.

Relative dependence is a stage that 'the infant can know about' (Winnicott, 1965b, p. 87), when the baby starts to come to terms with external reality. It is time for the mother to gradually introduce small doses of reality to the baby by allowing minor failures in her adaptations, so that the baby starts to be aware of its own dependence, the separateness of its mother and the reality that it is not omnipotent. It is also a stage where the baby learns about anxiety and loss when the mother is absent, and comes to understand the mother's personal and separate existence, 'and eventually the child comes to be able to believe in the parents' coming together which in fact led to his or her own conception' (Winnicott, 1965b, p. 90). Winnicott suggests that it is the development of the baby's intellect by the end of the first year that enables it to allow for failure in maternal adaptations. However, if the mothering is erratic and fails to adapt to the appropriate level of intellectual capacity of the baby, it is the mind of the baby that enables it to survive. In that case, thinking becomes a substitute for maternal care, and intellectualism becomes a defence.

The final 'towards independence' phase can never be completely accomplished, because a healthy individual is not isolated completely. On the contrary, the individual is always interdependent with the external environment, which in turn has a continuous outward movement from the mother to both parents, to family, to school, to wider society, and eventually to government in the outermost circle. In health, the ego holds the self, and it replaces the holding mother and gradually the wider outer social circle, which acts as a window to the outside world enabling the self to relate to external reality.

According to Winnicott, morality is a natural feature of human development and it does not need to be taught; indeed, guilt is a healthy sign of human development when the mother lets the baby experience its instinctual wishes and then allows it to make reparation for its primitive love impulse. Similar to Klein, Winnicott puts the origin of guilt in the first year of life. However, he reverses the relationship between Klein's guilt and reparation by stating that 'the guilt is not felt, but it lies dormant, or potential, and appears (as sadness or depressed mood) only if opportunity for reparation fails to turn up' (Winnicott, 1965b, p. 77). To Winnicott, the capacity for concern is a more developed form of guilt; guilt in the Kleinian sense is more negative and it is linked to anxiety and ambivalent feelings, but capacity for concern is more than reparation because it involves a sense of making a contribution to the other person; it 'implies further integration, and further growth, and relates in a positive way to the individual's sense of responsibility, especially in respect of relationships into which the instinctual drives have entered' (Winnicott, 1965b, p. 73).

The importance of play towards personality integration and creativity

Play is a central concept in Winnicott's theoretical framework, and being able to play is of fundamental importance to human development.

> It is play that is universal, and that belongs to health: playing facilitates growth and therefore health; playing leads into group relationships; playing can be a form of communication in psychotherapy; and, lastly, psychoanalysis has been developed as a highly specialized form of playing in the service of communication with oneself and others.
>
> (Winnicott, 1971a, p. 56)

Unlike Freud, Winnicott's play is not associated with erotic pleasure, even though play may arouse a certain level of anxiety. However, too much pleasure and anxiety can destroy playing.

Winnicott (1971a), divided play into three progressive stages: the first stage starts at the relative dependence period when the baby first experiences separation from its mother. In this first stage of play, it is important for the mother to encourage the baby to create a world that is coloured by the baby's phantasy as much as possible, a world that only exists in the potential space between the baby and the mother.

The second stage of play is when the baby has gained the capacity to play alone in the presence of someone. This capacity to be alone is a very important concept and it also shows how Winnicott differs from Klein, as he shifts psychoanalytic ideas from negative, anxiety-based psychopathology to positive potential. Klein suggests that the capacity to be alone is dependent on the existence of a good internal object, Winnicott does not deny the importance of the good internal object, but instead, he stresses that at least for a limited period of time, the baby does genuinely enjoy the experience of being alone in the presence of a reliable mother, who makes no demands. It is in this limited window that the baby can return to a period of un-integration, a period where sensations and impulses can be experienced as real and personal to the fullest, in the presence of a reliable mother.

The third and last stage of play is when the child allows the mother to introduce her playing and ideas into their play, ideas that have not originated from the child, and with the achievement of this stage, playing together in a relationship is made possible.

Winnicott regards playing as equivalent to art and religious practice in contributing towards the integration of personality, and no communication is possible with the external environment except through playing. Only in playing can the whole personality be used, aliveness be seen, and evidence of creativity be shown. In his theoretical explication of play and creativity, Winnicott managed to take one step further from Freud's anal psychosexual stage explanation of creativity as 'productions', to treating play, creativity and art as the only form of sublimation that combines the internal and external world, the pleasure and reality principle, into an intermediate, third area of experience in the 'potential space'.

Lev Vygotsky, a pioneering Russian psychologist, once said in a 1933 lecture on play that 'in play a child is always above his average age, above his daily behaviour; in play it is as though he were a head taller than himself. As in the focus of a magnifying glass, play contains all developmental tendencies in a condensed form; in play it is as though the child were trying to jump above the level of his normal behaviour' (Vygotsky, 1967). Consistent with the cardinal role placed on play, Winnicott has pushed it to further heights.

The task of mothering

The critical role of the mother in facilitating ego development

In Winnicott's developmental theory, the fundamental importance of the mother in facilitating the baby's ego integration and personality development is emphasised. He uses the term 'primary maternal preoccupation' (Winnicott, 1975, p. 302) to describe a period that occurs during pregnancy until a few weeks after the birth of the infant, when the mother develops an unusual state of heightened sensitivity and preoccupations with the needs of the infant, to the exclusion of her own needs and all other interests. Despite the intensity of this state, a failure of adaptation, it is temporary one and completely normal. Once this state is passed and the mother recovers from it, the memory of it is often repressed. However, not all women can enter the state of primary maternal preoccupation, and when that happens, the baby's development will be affected (Winnicott, 1975).

To Winnicott, mothering is certainly special but it is also an innate ability that can be performed well by an 'ordinary devoted mother' (Winnicott, 1988a, pp. 3–14), who has been a baby herself before, so her skills come naturally without needing to learn from books or doctors, paediatricians, or midwives. The role of this 'ordinary devoted mother' is to be a 'good enough' mother in order to provide a holding environment that facilitates the natural developmental process of the baby (Winnicott, 1965b). 'Good enough' in Winnicott's definition does not mean mediocrity or having any form of compromise: there does exist a group of 'not-good-enough' mothers who repeatedly fail to meet the baby's needs which is a form of environmental impingement that leads to compliance and premature development of the false self (Winnicott, 1965a).

Unlike Klein who describes the baby's perception of its mother as both the 'good breast' that provides and satisfies and the 'bad breast' that frustrates, Winnicott further expands Klein's construct by incorporating the importance of the environment. He describes the two different functions, rather than perceptions or experiences as Klein did, of the mother as an 'object mother', who satisfies the needs as well as contains the hate of the infant, and as an 'environmental mother', who holds the baby physically as well as emotionally before the boundaries of time and space are firmly established within the infant. This maternal holding also protects the baby from external environmental impingements, including the frustrations of the mother in handling the infant (Winnicott, 1964). This early holding gradually evolves into an ego-support that is required in adulthood, when there is excessive deprivation or stress.

In 'Mirror-role of mother and family in child development', explicates two important functions of the mother. First, during the mothering process, she serves as a mirror for the baby in order to see itself, and for the mother to see what she looks like to the baby, through a reflection of herself in its eyes. A 'good enough mother' is able to facilitate the following sequence of perceptions by the baby: 'When I look I am seen, so I exist. I can now afford to look and see. I now look creatively and what I apperceive I also perceive. In fact I take care not to see what is not there to be seen (unless I am tired)' (Winnicott, 1971a, p. 154). Winnicott's mirror is very different from Lacan's, which focuses solely on the baby's discovery of the self in the mirror (the mother's eyes), whereas in Winnicott's framework what the baby sees is a comprehensive experience of the self and a reflection of the self in the mirror. Second, the mother needs to continuously adapt to the needs of the baby; from complete adaptation during the baby's absolute dependence stage, and repeatedly meeting the needs of the baby in order to facilitate the experience of an illusion of omnipotence, to the gradual introduction of small doses of reality to disillusion the baby via failing to adapt to all its needs during the relative dependence stage. Winnicott asserted that the ability to fail to adapt is vital as 'a mother who cannot gradually fail on this matter of sensitive adaptation is failing in another sense; she is failing (because of her own immaturity or her own anxieties) to give her infant reasons for anger' (Winnicott, 1965b, p. 87). Through complete adaptation, it is the mother who first provides the baby with an 'illusion' that it has created the breast, just at the right moment when it needs nourishment. Through this repeated 'creation' of the breast, the baby gradually develops an expectation and confidence that it can find any objects of desire anytime, anywhere, in a magical way. As the baby builds up memories of the image of the breast, it can gradually tolerate the absence of the breast because the baby knows that it can magically create the breast. This is the moment where the mother can start to gradually disillusion the baby by introducing small doses of reality and by failing to adapt, in line with the infant's growing ability to tolerate her absence and failure, which also provides the necessary groundwork for weaning at a later stage.

It is worth mentioning here that 'illusion' is an essential concept in Winnicott's theoretical construct, and this is where one can see another radical departure from, if not a complete break from Freud's conception of 'illusion'. To Freud, 'illusion' has a negative connotation and is linked to the pathology and neurosis that needs to be eliminated in the reality testing process. On the contrary, Winnicott attaches a positive meaning to 'illusion' and links it to creativity and its value as an inseparable factor in human development from infancy to adulthood. Winnicott indicates that the movement between illusion and disillusion persists throughout life, that 'the task of reality-acceptance is never completed, that no human being is free from the strain of relating inner and outer reality, and that relief from this strain is provided by an intermediate area of experience which is not challenged (arts, religion, etc.)' (Winnicott, 1975, p. 240). Winnicott's concept of the transitional object, which I will go on to outline, is something that belongs to this intermediate area.

In contrast to Freud's view of illusion, which is regarded as erroneous thinking that is emotionally charged by early wish-fulfilment desire and thus to be replaced by reality testing and rational thought (Freud, 1927), Winnicott transforms the term 'illusion' radically, by attributing a positive nature to it, and giving it a positive place in human development. Winnicott suggests that illusion is instrumental in permitting the child to gradually relate to the outside world. By 'creating' the world through illusion, the child is gradually being disillusioned by the mother as she slowly introduces external reality in small doses to the child. When that happens, a different illusion is formed, and the cycle continues. The capacity for illusion remains a positive trait for the developing child, as it is a means for it to experience and assimilate new situations throughout life. In order to extend Winnicott's thinking one step further, since we all live in a world of shared illusions, absolute reality is, in fact, an unknown. This is in line with Bion's 'O', which denotes the absolute truth that cannot be known (Bion, 1977).

Winnicott points out that the key difference between illusion and delusion is that an illusion can be shared with others and it can change as new experiences and reality impinge, whereas a delusion is a personal reality that one imposes upon others. Winnicott's conceptualisation of delusion can be regarded as similar to Freud's, in which Freud regards delusion as a belief that is highly improbable and incompatible with what we can observe in objective reality, and unlike the illusion that is religion, the illusion that is psychoanalysis is open to change (Freud, 1927). Usuelli (1972) observes that Freud's idea of transference, when a patient treats the analyst as if he were a figure from the past, may be classified as illusionary. To a certain extent, the therapeutic relationship is also a shared illusion that the therapist participates in, in search of understanding, insight, and change. The therapy session represents a transitional space where new experiences and insights are discovered, and is eventually, though not entirely relinquished.

Transitional objects and transitional phenomenon

The transitional object is a different type of illusion and it belongs to the stage during and after weaning, between the ages of four to twelve months. As the infant begins to separate 'me' from 'not me', it makes use of the transitional object to bridge the subjective and objective experience, which belongs neither to the baby nor the mother, but to an intermediate area between the internal and the external worlds. For the infant, the transitional object is a part of itself, like a mouth or a breast.

Perhaps the easiest way to understand the complex idea of the transitional object is to refer to the *Peanuts* comic strip character, Linus, created by Charles Schulz. Linus is the middle child of the van Pelt family, he is portrayed by Schulz as the strip's intellectual, a deep thinker who is bright yet fragile. Linus is always seen sucking his thumb while clinging to a blanket, which represents the epitome of security. In 1955, Winnicott wrote to Charles Schulz seeking permission to reproduce an image of Linus sucking his thumb and clinging to his security blanket as an example of the transitional object which was to be described in his forthcoming book (Winnicott, 1955b).

The transitional object belongs to an intermediate experience therefore one should never ask the infant 'did you conceive of this or was it presented to you from without?' (Winnicott, 1975, p. 235). The object is discovered or created by the infant, and regarded as an inseparable part of it, that is, between the thumb and an external object. The transitional object is likely to be something soft and pliable, something readily available and within easy reach of the baby, for example, a piece of wool pulled from a blanket or a napkin, so in a way, while it is indirectly provided by the mother, it is never deliberately offered by the mother, because it is simply impossible for the mother to provide a transitional object to the baby. What she can provide is only a comforter, a mother substitute that is regarded by the baby as less important than the mother herself.

The transitional object is the infant's first possession, and each infant has its unique way of creating the first possession. The infant believes that it has created the transitional object, and this belief in the creation process is important as it is a necessary illusion of omnipotence. This necessary developmental journey leads to the use of illusion, the use of symbols, and the use of an object.

Winnicott lists seven special qualities in the relationship between the infant and his transitional object:

1. The infant assumes rights over the object, and we agree to this assumption. Nevertheless some abrogation of omnipotence is a feature from the start.
2. The object is affectionately cuddled as well as excitedly loved and mutilated.
3. It must never change, unless changed by the infant.
4. It must survive instinctual loving, and also hating, and, if it be a feature, pure aggression.
5. Yet it must seem to the infant to give warmth, or to move, or to have texture, or to do something that seems to show it has a vitality or reality of its own.

6. It comes from without from our point of view, but not so from the point of view of the baby. Neither does it come from within; it is not a hallucination.

7. Its fate is to be gradually allowed to be decathected, so that in the course of years it becomes not so much forgotten as relegated to limbo. By this we mean that in health the transitional object does not 'go inside', nor does the feeling about it necessarily undergo repression. It is not forgotten and it is not mourned. It loses its meaning, and this is because the transitional phenomena have become diffused, and have become spread out over the whole intermediate territory between the 'inner psychic reality' and 'the external world as perceived by two persons in common', that is to say, over the whole cultural field.

(Winnicott, 1953, p. 91)

Closely linked to the transitional object is the idea of potential space or transitional phenomena (Winnicott, 1971a). This is an intermediate area between the subjective inner reality and objective external shared reality, a dimension of living that belongs to neither an internal nor external reality. It cannot be challenged because we do not know whether it is created by the baby, or whether it contains some of the perceived reality. This intermediate area is a state that parents would allow the baby to be in during childhood, and that society would permit in adulthood, especially when it gradually widens out over time in the intense experience of the areas of arts, religion, imaginative living, and creative scientific work, as long as the person in this state does not force others to share the same personal illusion with him.

Winnicott suggests that there is a natural and innate propensity for healthy human development towards maturity. This includes physical and emotional maturity, as well as moral codes and other cultural phenomena. These cannot be taught to the baby, nor can they be hurried. The role of the mother is to provide a facilitating environment in order to encourage her infant, not to dominate it's natural creative growth and impose her values onto it. Similarly, the adolescent needs to discover his own maturation, including his need to challenge and metaphorically murder his parents, and what the parents need to do is to endure and survive no matter how violent the attacks are (Winnicott, 1971).

According to Winnicott, transitional phenomena and the transitional object are the basis of initiation of experience and object relations of the infant, therefore they are signs of healthy development, and are made possible by the presence of a 'good enough mother', who, in a state of 'primary maternal preoccupation', continuously adapts to the needs of the infant by gradually introducing appropriate doses of an external reality to it. This is achieved by the creation of a 'holding environment' and an illusion that reinforces the infant's feelings of omnipotence, an illusion that the infant is capable of creating an outer reality that can relieve instinctual tension, and where the breast is part of the infant's creation and is therefore under its magical control. If this illusion can be successfully established, a good internal object is created and the 'good enough mother' can begin to gradually disillusion the infant by introducing small doses of the world to the infant, as its capacity to tolerate frustration increases over time.

Furthermore, Winnicott (1965a, cited in Abram, 2007, p. 223, pp. 243–244) also postulates that apart from the 'good enough mother', there is another group of 'not-good-enough mothers', which can be sub-divided into three different types. The first one is the 'psychotic mother', who is in a state of 'pathological preoccupation', in which she is able to adapt to the infant's need at the beginning, but fails to acknowledge the infant's need to separate from her later on, so she continues to identify with the infant for too long. Another type is the 'mother who cannot surrender to primary maternal preoccupation', probably because she is depressed or preoccupied. The final type is the 'tantalising mother', who is highly inconsistent in her handling of the infant and oscillates between holding and dropping: this type of mother is the most damaging to the ego development of the infant. The 'not-good-enough' mothers are the root of maternal failure, as they force the infant to find a way to protect its illusion of fleeting omnipotence by developing a pathological, false, compliant self, which in turn leads to an ego distortion and schizoid characteristics in later life. Winnicott's view is consistent with Milner (1952), who suggested that maternal failure is a precursor to premature ego development and a disturbed illusionary period. Because of this disturbance, the ego is forced into precocious differentiation between the bad and the good object, and the individual can go through life searching for the valuable 'resting place' of illusion that they missed in their early childhood.

Winnicott writes in a beautiful and poetic way. His spontaneous style and his fondness for using paradoxes, and playing with words and ideas, make his work unique in the academic world. As a result of this highly creative thinking and writing style, his work is best suited as an inspiration for other theorists, both within and outside of the psychoanalytic field. Like any other psychoanalytic concept, Winnicott's ideas need to be validated thoroughly and carefully. As Jacobs suggests:

> ... those who are able to conduct quantifiable research are in a position to see how much of what he writes is verifiable. Those whose interest lies in the world of ideas can pursue the internal logic of psychoanalytic discourse. Those who seek to apply his ideas to practice might test out how transferable they are to their own situations. All such attempts demonstrate the catalytic effect Winnicott has on theory and practice.
>
> (Jacobs, 1995, p. 120)

The 'catalytic effect' may be seen in the wide-ranging literature written on transitional object and phenomena after the release of Winnicott's 1953 paper, 'Transitional objects and transitional phenomena – a study of the first not-me possession'. A PEP-Web subject search on the 'transitional object' and 'transitional phenomena' returned 83 hits, whereas a content search resulted in over 300 hits. The psychoanalytic literature on transitional objects and phenomena after Winnicott range from theoretical and clinical validations, elaboration on the nature of a transitional object, attempts at expanding or integrating Winnicott's idea of transitional objects and phenomena, to applications of these ideas in clinical settings and to the exploration in art and culture.

Theoretical and clinical validations of a transitional object and phenomena:

- Some writers provided supporting evidence on the existence of transitional phenomena (Kahne, 1967; Athanassiou, 1991; Burch, 1993).
- Stevenson & Winnicott (1954) found that a transitional object was more common amongst children living with their families than those in residential nurseries, and the finding was supported by Provence and Lipton (1962).
- Gaddini and Gaddini (1970) conducted the first systematic study of the transitional object based on maternal interviews in Italy, and found that, compared to urban children, rural children had a significantly lower incidence of having a transitional object, which could be explained by the greater physical contact between the rural children and their mothers, making it less necessary for them to acquire a transitional object as a symbol of their mothers.
- Gaddini and Gaddini's (1970) study was subsequently replicated by Hong and Townes (1976) with American and Korean children. They found that the incidence of a transitional object was highest in the American children, followed by Korean children who lived in America, and lowest amongst Korean children living in Korea.
- Hong and Townes' (1976) finding was consistent with Gaddini and Gaddini's (1970), in which the incidence of a transitional object attachment was higher when the duration of breastfeeding was shorter, and vice versa.
- By observing 40 infants ranging from 11 to 19 months old, Parker (1979) classified the infants with and without transitional objects into three attachment groups, as defined by Ainsworth and Wittig's Strange Situation Test (1969), including the securely attached group, the anxious-ambivalent insecurely attached group, and the anxious-avoidant insecurely attached group. Parker found that almost all the infants amongst the anxious-avoidant insecurely attached group had no transitional objects, and that infants with transitional objects were weaned earlier, cried less during separations, and were able to be more independent of their mothers when handled by them. On the contrary, mothers of infants without transitional objects encouraged a more prolonged dependence on themselves by the infants.
- Parker's findings also support the findings of Gaddini and Gaddini (1970) and Hong and Townes (1976) that children who had more close contact with their mothers had a lower incidence of transitional objects.
- Busch (1974), Busch and McKnight (1973, 1977), and Busch et al. (1973) found a higher incidence of transitional objects amongst families with a higher education and upper-middle socioeconomic class.
- Brody and Axelrad (1970, 1978) did a longitudinal study observing 131 infants and interviewed their mothers regularly during the first year, followed by annual interviews for seven years. They found that, compared to

the lower-middle and below classes, significantly more children of middle and above socioeconomic status had transitional objects, supporting the findings of Gaddini and Gaddini (1970), Hong and Townes (1976), and Busch and McKnight (1973, 1977).

- Horton et al. (1974) found that the majority of the 19 men in his study, who had severe personality disorders, had poor object relations, and did not have any transitional object in their childhood, indicating that there seems to be value in the personality and emotional development in the childhood possession of a transitional object, although excessive attachment could be seen as a diagnostic sign for schizophrenia in adulthood (Horton, 1977).

Despite the challenges to Winnicott's concept of transitional objects and transitional phenomena, one cannot deny the similarity between the transitional phenomena and the transference reactions in therapy, because the patient finds himself feeling a strong emotion towards the therapist as if the therapist were someone significant in the patient's childhood, and at the same time the patient is very clear on the present reality and of the identity of the therapist. This is similar to Freud's view on transference, that 'transference … creates an intermediate region between illness and real life through which transition from one to the other is made' (Freud, 1914, p. 154).

Most of the transitional object and transitional phenomena literature studies after Winnicott focused on confirming or rejecting the existence of such phenomena, or applying the concepts to the understanding of psychopathology and clinical techniques, or extending the concepts, or integrating them with other existing psychoanalytical frameworks, and more importantly, on the study of the re-emergence of an infantile transitional object in adulthood.

On the nature of a transitional object:

- Fintzy (1971) explored the evolution and shifting change in the choice of a transitional object in a borderline child.
- Busch (1974) examined how the attachment to transitional objects developed and their respective functions.
- Greenacre (1969, 1970) and Roiphe and Galenson (1975) examined the similarities and differences between a transitional object and the fetish.
- Sloate (2008) indicated that the bulimic patients' self-infliction was more closely linked to the use of food or their bodies as a fetish object instead of a transitional object.
- Davidson (1976) investigated the difference between a transitional object, and symbols and transference.

Expanding or integrating Winnicott's theory:

*   Stevenson & Winnicott (1954) suggested that there are two types of transitional objects that a child becomes attached to at two distinct times in its life, i.e. the first year and the second year respectively.
*   Drawing on Greenson's (1954) discovery on the humming sensation and Winnicott's (1953) view on the auditory component of transitional phenomena, McDonald (1970) hypothesised the existence of a 'transitional tune' as an important early experience to facilitate the development of some musicians.
*   Busch and McKnight (1977) emphasised that the first transitional object should be distinguished from the second transitional object, the fetish object, objects that have a different locus and origin, and objects that are used to meet a direct libidinal need.
*   Bollas (1979) suggested that the first object or the mother can be conceived of as a 'transformational object', who transforms the self-experience of the infant from symbiotic relating to object representation, and that a transitional object is the heir to the transformational phase when the transformational process is displaced by the transitional object from the mother-environment into other subjective-objects.
*   Summers (1999) discussed how Winnicott's transitional space concept transformed the task of psychoanalyst from that of offering interpretation, to one of adaptation.
*   Vivona (2000) postulated the existence of a 'post-oedipal transitional object', as opposed to the 'pre-oedipal transitional object' formulated by Winnicott and asserted that it helps create an adult mind with mature psychological capacities to harbour neurotic conflicts.
*   Gaddini (2003) argued that 'precursor objects' precede transitional objects.
*   LaMothe (2005) reformulated Winnicott's 'potential space' into four interrelated dialectical processes of 'surrender-generation', 'recognition-negotiation', 'care-quiescence', and 'disruption-repair'.

Theoretical integration of transitional objects and transitional phenomena with other psychoanalytic concepts:

*   Tolpin (1971) applied the concept of Kohut's 'transmuting internalisation' (Kohut, 1975) in order to delineate the role of a transitional object in ego development.

- Hong (1978) reviewed psychoanalytic, experimental, ethological and cross-cultural studies of transitional phenomena, and attempted a theoretical integration and classification of transitional phenomena.
- Ogden (1985) re-articulated the concept of 'potential space' as a state of mind based on a series of opposing relationships, e.g. between phantasy and reality, 'me' and 'not me', symbol and symbolised.
- Adler (1989) regarded the designed ambiguous nature of a psychoanalytic session as a re-creation of transitional phenomena that promotes the capacity for a creative use of illusion and play.
- Civin and Lombardi (1990) attempted to synthesise Freud's concept of the 'preconscious' and Winnicott's concept of 'potential space'.
- Pedder (1992) linked psychotherapy and the experience in the theatre to transitional space.
- Kuriloff (1998) compared Winnicott's transitional space with Sullivan's interpersonal model.
- Bram and Gabbard (2001) explored the connection between 'potential space' and reflective functioning.
- Tibon (2005) conducted a quantitative study to explore the similarity between psychosomatics and psychosis using Winnicott's idea on 'potential space'.
- Chatterji (2009) explored the conceptual similarities between Winnicott's transitional phenomena and D. H. Lawrence's theoretical framework on the unconscious.

Applications of a transitional object and phenomena in clinical settings to understand psychopathology:

- Modell (1963) and Cooper & Adler (1990) applied the concept of a transitional object to analyse borderline patients.
- Volkan and Kavanaugh (1978) used it to analyse narcissistic patients.
- Straetz (1976) applied it to the understanding of a psychopathologic origin of adolescent behaviour.
- Downey (1978) used the idea of transitional phenomena in an adolescent analysis to identify the presence of transference neurosis.
- Ogden (1985) explored the implications on psychopathology of potential space and divided patients into three groups depending on their relationship with phantasy and reality. The first group is defined as having a sense of reality engulfed by phantasy. These are the borderline patients operating on the basis of symbolic equations. The second group is composed of those who use reality as a defence against phantasy. This is the group where there is a foreclosure of imagination. The third group is composed

of those who dissociate phantasy from reality. This is a state of non-experience, as meanings are not created. This is when there is a foreclosure of both reality and phantasy.

- Dithrich (1991) connected pathological lying to a potential space.
- Dimen (1991) explored the role of transitional space in transference and counter-transference, when both the patient and the analyst alternate between being gendered and being gender-free.
- Goldman (1996) examined the dynamics of 'potential space' generated in the therapeutic sessions.
- Pizer (1996) and Elkind (2002) explored clinical techniques that leverage on the therapeutic use of transitional space.
- Ehrenberg (1976) developed the 'intimate edge' technique in order to enhance the capacity for a creative and imaginative experience in the transitional phenomena in a therapeutic relationship.
- Resch et al. (1988) attempted a therapeutic re-construction of a transitional object for a ten-year-old girl, which proved to be effective in facilitating significant development in symbolic functioning.
- Os (1991) discussed the internalisation of the analyst and the analytic relation, and the creation and subsequent internalisation of the transitional object in therapy.
- Mann (1998) demonstrated how the clinical use of dreams facilitated the creation of transitional space and strengthened the ego capacity to do integration work within that space.
- Teitelbaum (2003) discussed how the analyst was used as a transitional object in a psychoanalytic therapy in order to facilitate therapeutic progress.

Exploration of the role of transitional phenomena in art and culture:

- Modell (1970) and Hopkins (2002) connected the art piece and art creation process to the development of 'potential space' shared between the artists and the recipients.
- Hanchett (1976) explored the connection between transitional phenomena and cultural and social anthropology.
- Miller (1992) explored the common 'potential space' between writers and their readers.
- Jemstedt (2000) built on Winnicott and Bion's theories and postulated that creativity and creative living is the result of the development of inner space and 'potential space'.
- Grandy and Tuber (2009) used the metaphors of transitioning into an imaginary space in children's literature in order to explore variations in the affective quality of 'potential space'.

Father and the wider family

Compared to the mother, Winnicott has placed significantly less emphasis on the role of the father, for which he is often criticised as undermining the importance of the father. To Winnicott, the father 'can help provide a space ... properly protected by her man, the mother is saved from having to turn outwards to deal with her surroundings at the time when she is wanting to turn inwards' (Winnicott, 1964, p. 25). Therefore, the role of the father is to provide a secure environment, both physically and emotionally, for the mother in order to allow her to go into the primary maternal preoccupation state, and dedicate her whole self to providing a facilitating environment for the infant during the entire development process. Specifically, this secure environment includes first, social and financial security through his relationship with the mother; second, moral support by reinforcing the mother's authority and representing a symbol of law and order, as 'he does not have to be there all the time to do this, but he has to turn up often enough for the child to feel that he is real and alive' (Winnicott, 1964, p. 115); third, the father provides a role model for men, how they should behave by going to work each morning and returning at night, although Winnicott says that 'it is mother's responsibility to send father and daughter, or father and son, out together for an expedition now and again' (Winnicott, 1964, p. 118). Finally, Winnicott mentions that the father assists in the process of separation between the baby and the mother through a 'to-and-fro' experience, where the baby moves between the parents and the extended family (Winnicott, 1986).

Winnicott's strengths lie in his acute observation of the early mother-infant relationship. He did not seem to be interested in the mother and child relationship after the first six months, although he saw children of all ages in his practice. Central to his work is the relationship of the mother-infant nursing couple, which is also the focus of major criticism of his having a one-sided emphasis on the mother while neglecting the role the father plays in the development of the child. For example, in *Playing and reality* (1971a), there are only three mentions of the word 'father', perhaps indicating a lack of interest in the paternal role (Rycroft, 1985; Samuels, 1993).

In Winnicott's model, the father always plays a supportive role in facilitating a secure environment to the mother, allowing her to enter the primary maternal preoccupation mode at the beginning of the infant's life. Afterwards, the father provides an example of a separate person to the infant, and gradually develops into the traditional Oedipal role. Winnicott said that infant care 'can be done well by only one person' (Winnicott, 1964, p. 24). However, he did note that it was possible for the father to play the role of the mother, but he performs not exactly the role of the father but rather that of a mother substitute (Winnicott, 1965a). This view is a significant departure from the Kleinian one, which suggested that the father protects the child from the mother, and the mother from the child, so the father's support is perceived by the child as instrumental in restoring the emotional health of the mother after the baby's phantasised attack on her (Segal, 1992).

What can go wrong in the developmental process?

Psychopathology

Winnicott's developmental model is a positive one, and he emphasises that normal development in the infant is innate. The importance of the mother lies in providing a good enough holding environment by continually adapting to the needs of the baby according to its developmental stage, through which continuity and a going-on being is being preserved, and the individual is able to feel real and to experience an age-appropriate emotional life. Unlike Freud and Klein, Winnicott does not appear to be very interested in the psychopathology and anxieties of human development. He did write about the false self, which is a defence developed to ward off environmental impingements. He also attributes a psychotic illness to an environmental failure in facilitating the natural maturational process. This type of failure is called 'privation' (Winnicott, 1965b, p. 226), where developmental success has never been achieved. Privation is to be distinguished from 'deprivation', which means that a failure occurs after a certain development success has been accomplished. It is associated with an 'antisocial tendency' (Winnicott, 1975) such as stealing and destructiveness, which can be found in normal individuals. Winnicott suggests that an antisocial tendency needs to be treated by the provision of proper childcare to enable the child to experiment again with its id impulses (Winnicott, 1975, p. 315).

In Winnicott's maturational development theory, there is a clear parallel between the growth of the baby and the journey towards an effective psychoanalytic therapy, and between the role of the mother in providing a holding environment, and the role of the psychotherapist in providing space and boundaries so that trust can be experienced in the therapeutic relationship. Primary maternal preoccupation can be compared to the therapist's attentive listening via their evenly suspended attention during therapy, and via maternal holding with sensitive adaptations to how the therapist carefully allows the patient to experience the internal and external worlds in small doses in a safe environment, protecting from too much and encouraging access when appropriate. Development can only take place at the pace selected by the infant, and in a therapeutic situation, the therapist practises with extreme care how much in the way of interpretation he offers. Preferably, the therapist would allow the patient to explore and reveal an interpretation by himself, as if it is created by him (Winnicott, 1971a). One very refreshing view from Winnicott is that a good technique may facilitate a corrective experience of therapy, but what is more important is that the small failures of therapists that would trigger hatred in the patient which would in turn help to bring original environmental failures into the transference relationship. When this happens, it is imperative for the therapist to survive and stay alive, so in a way the therapist's failure succeeds in helping the patient develop and recover. According to Winnicott, the objective of therapy is to enable the patient to break free from their false self, and progress towards the development of a less compliant and more integrated true self and personal core (Winnicott, 1975).

Unlike Freud and Klein, who focused on developing grand theories such as Freud's instinct theory, the unconscious, the centrality of sexuality, and the tripartite structure of the mind and the personality, or Klein's notions of paranoid-schizoid and depressive positions, Winnicott's objective was to provide insight into the stages of human development that precede object relations and published many papers to support his observations.

Winnicott's positive view of human nature is in sharp contrast to Freud and Klein's somewhat bleak and disillusioned view of humanity. Winnicott rejects Freud's death instinct, and he uses 'concern' to replace 'guilt' to mean that the infant develops a sense of concern towards its mother for providing a holding environment, rather than experiencing guilt, as in Klein's theoretical construct. Moreover, Klein interprets joy as a manic defence, whereas Winnicott sees joy and creativity as an inseparable part of natural human experience, and he also disagrees with the Kleinian notion of projection, where the infant projects the undesirable part of itself onto people outside (Eigen, 1981).

There has been some concern over Winnicott's extreme optimism towards humanity in his theories, and that he may not have sufficiently taken into consideration the ambivalence of human relationships. In fact, Winnicott's emphasis on positive features is in marked contrast to the Freudian and Kleinian approaches of treating all positives with extreme caution, and of treating it as a defence against aggression and destructiveness.

Chapter 8

What is D. W. Winnicott's view on smoking addiction?

The reappearance of an infantile transitional object in adulthood

From the date of publication, 1953 to 2022, Winnicott's 'Transitional objects and transitional phenomena' has the highest search volume on PEP-Web, and it is also the second most cited paper with 1,323 cumulative citations, slightly below Klein's 'Notes on some schizoid mechanisms' (1946) with 1,543 citations, and higher than Bion's 'Attacks on linking' (1959) with 979 citations.

Winnicott holds that transitional objects typically begin to appear from four-to-six to eight-to-twelve months: '… in health the transitional object doesn't not "go inside" nor does the feeling about it necessarily undergo repression. It is not forgotten and it is not mourned. It loses meaning, and this is because the transitional phenomena have become diffused, have become spread out over the whole intermediate territory between "inner psychic reality" and "the external world as perceived by two persons in common", that is to say, over the whole cultural field'. He concludes that 'An infant's transitional object ordinarily becomes gradually decathected, especially as cultural interests develop' (Winnicott, 1953, p. 91).

In psychopathology:

Addiction can be stated in terms of regression to the early stage at which the transitional phenomena are unchallenged.

Fetish can be described in terms of a persistence of a specific object or type of object dating from infantile experience in the transitional field, linked with the delusion of a maternal phallus.

Pseudologia and thieving can be described in terms of an individual's unconscious urge to bridge a gap in continuity of experience in respect of a transitional object.

(Winnicott, 1953, p. 97)

After mentioning the relationship between the regressive appearance of transitional phenomenon and addiction, Winnicott did not further elaborate his views on addiction. In the original version of his 1953 paper, presented in a meeting attended

DOI: 10.4324/9781003329077-12

by members of the British Psychoanalytic Society on 30 May 1951, Winnicott included a few paragraphs about the abnormalities on the development of transitional objects but these were subsequently removed in revisions of the same work in 1953, 1958, and 1971 respectively:

> Abnormalities. The main abnormality, I suggest, arises out of discontinuity of experience relative to transitional objects and phenomena. As a result there is either no transitional object or else an exaggeration of the dependence on the original transitional object with limitation of spread of interests. I attempt to explain this in Part III, but at this point I wish to refer to one clinical type, the anti-social child, typically a thief.
>
> Psychology of Stealing. The thief is trying (amongst other things), to fill the gap in experience of transitional objects. While he has hope he steals. He seeks the affectionate relationship which belongs to transitional phenomena. In the lying that goes with stealing is hidden the claim that a story can be both fantasy and fact.
>
> The aetiology of thieving cannot, in fact, be fully worked out expect on a basis of the thief's attempt to recover lost transitional phenomena. It must be remembered that the delinquent is not depressed or mad when delinquent, though depression or madness may in some cases be the alternatives to anti-social behaviour.
>
> (Winnicott, 1951, cited in Caldwell & Robinson, 2016, pp. 450–451)

However, Winnicott did not further elaborate on the idea around 'no transitional object or else an exaggeration of the dependence on the original transitional object with limitation of spread of interests' in 'Part III', which is more focused on explaining the differences between transitional object and Klein's internal object.

In the absence of further explication on the relationship between transitional objects and addiction, what we can infer from Winnicott's 1953 paper is that a transitional object is not always as transitional as its name suggests, it can remain for a longer period of time in early childhood to provide a regressive comfort, especially when the child is confronted by stress. In fact, since 1953, a number of studies have shown that instead of being given up in later life, an infantile transitional object can reappear in later adult life in a regressed form, and that other symptoms and rituals are developed as a substitution of the regressed infantile transitional object until it is finally given up.

Reappearance of infantile transitional object in a regressed form

- Fink (1962) regarded the pacifier as a transitional object.
- Schlierf (1983) examined how prescribed medication was used as a transitional object, and how such insight could contribute to the understanding of the therapist being used as an ego-supportive entity and a magical omnipotent object in patients with anxiety neurosis.

- Giovacchini (1984, 1987) discussed how children were used as transitional objects by their mothers, leading to a fixation of emotional development in the transitional space and ego, as well as character defects in their adulthood.
- Turkel (1998) linked female compulsive eating and dieting to how girls were raised through distorted and stereotyped transitional objects.
- Coppolillo (1967) reported a young adult using their psychotically depressed mother as a transitional object after she intervened in their use of a transitional object when they were five years old. The patient even perceived the analyst and the analysis itself as transitional objects during his treatment.
- In Kafka's (1969) study, a patient treated his own body as a transitional object and said that he had a sensation of becoming alive, as if he was protected by a security blanket, when he felt the blood flowing out onto his body from the cuts he inflicted himself.
- McDonald (1970) asserted that lullabies have a quality of being a transitional object because of the connection between these songs and childhood, leading to the child's belief that the lullabies are created by it and can be reproduced by it at will. Parish (1978) further expanded McDonald's idea by saying that any thought or object could serve as a transitional object to bridge the internal psychic world and the external reality.
- Gay and Hyson (1976) observed that when confronted with stress, their five-year-old respondents picked up their infantile transitional objects immediately and displayed increased regressive behaviours during the time when they were holding their transitional objects. According to normal development progress, children after the age of two or three should be able to tolerate the temporary loss of a loved object through diverting their energy towards the use of more developed symbolic objects for self-soothing. The fact that children of the age of five in Gay and Hyson's study are still dependent on their infantile transitional objects suggests a lack of an age-appropriate capacity to use symbolised objects, and if this is reinforced by the prolonged attachment to infantile transitional objects, neurotic withdrawal may be further strengthened. Gay and Hyson's finding is consistent with Fintzy's (1971) finding where he reported a persistent use of transitional objects as a magical blanket in a borderline child of five years old. On that, Brody (1980) also pointed out that a persistent attachment to the transitional objects during waking hours beyond two years old may reflect weakness and immaturity in ego development, resulting in the child's inability to direct energy to age-appropriate interests and activities.
- Downey (1978) suggested that there is a high level of resemblance between some adolescent behaviours and the use of infantile transitional

objects. For instance, the adolescent's wish for clothes versus the infant's wish to attract or disgust parents, the adolescent's fondness of listening to loud music versus the infant's use of early noisy toys, and the adolescent's treatments of their possessions and therapy versus the infant's ambivalent use of transitional objects. Downey argued that these behaviours suggested that the adolescent was trying to re-create his early internal and external worlds through music and his current possessions for a self-soothing purpose.

- Grolnick and Lengyel (1978) observed the parallel between the infantile use of a transitional object to overcome separation anxiety before going to sleep, and the Etruscan funerary symbols that are used to defend against the anxiety of death.
- Volkan and Kavanaugh (1978) observed that borderline patients used their cats as a regressed infantile transitional object and established similar object relations with the cats.
- Dinnage (1978) suggested that Freud's antiquities were his regressed form of infantile transitional objects.
- Sugarman and Kurash (1982a) examined the use of marijuana as a transitional object by the borderline adolescent to temporarily transcend developmental limitations and to increase subjective experience of a heightened level of cognitive functioning.
- In an attempt to examine the relationship between early traumatic object relations and addiction, Miller (2002) argued that the root cause of drug addiction can be explained by approaching a needle as a transitional object.

Smoking addiction is a regression to the infantile bliss of reunion with one's mother

After reviewing the index on 'addiction', 'perverse transitional object', and 'pathological transitional object' in the 12-volume *Collected works of D. W. Winnicott* (Caldwell and Taylor Robinson, 2017), one very interesting and relevant report was found. In 'Comments on the report of the committee on punishment in prisons and borstals', Winnicott states that:

> … one does not have to be a psychoanalyst to know that smoking is not just something done for pleasure. It is something which has a very great importance in the lives of many people, and which cannot be given up without substitution of something else. Smoking can be vitally important to individuals, especially when there is widespread hopelessness in a community. The psychoanalyst is able to watch at close quarters the use of tobacco and indeed there is a great

deal of research to be done on this subject before it can be properly understood. Without waiting for clear understanding, it is possible already to state that smoking is one of the ways in which individuals can just hold on to sanity, when without smoking and especially if alcohol and other drugs are withheld, the sense of reality is lost and the personality tends to disintegrate. There is of course a great deal more in smoking than this, but I think it should be appreciated by those who deal with the subject of smoking in prisons that the fact that so much trafficking in tobacco goes on in spite of all regulations and in spite of every possible effort on the part of the authorities to curb it, confirms one theory, which is that criminals are on the whole in a state of great distress and a constant fear of madness.

(Winnicott, 1984 in Caldwell & Taylor Robinson, 2017, pp. 274–275)

This is very similar to the observed high usage of cigarettes amongst patients with mental disorders in psychiatric hospitals. For instance, in the UK, 44 per cent of people with psychotic disorders living in community settings were smokers, of which 27 per cent were heavy smokers (O'Brien et al., 2002). Moreover, among those with severe mental illness who used inpatient services, up to 70 per cent were smokers (Coulthard et al., 2002), and around half of those smoked heavily (Meltzer, 1996). R. D. Hinshelwood (Personal communication), also observed that instead of speaking to each other, many psychiatric patients used cigarettes to form social connections with each other. This indicates that rather than connecting with others via cultural activities, disadvantaged people may use cigarettes as a physical, bodily, and concrete object to connect with each other.

This observation fits with Winnicott's view that smoking is how this group of disadvantaged people, who are in a state of hopelessness, constant distress and fear of madness, 'hold on to sanity' in an attempt to prevent a disintegration of personality and a complete loss of reality. However, these attempts do not seem to be successful, as is evident in the habit of smoking, and it does seem that some kind of false self-manifestation must keep repeating itself through the continued use of cigarettes. Unfortunately, while stating in the 1951 report that 'there is a great deal of research to be done on this subject (smoking addiction) before it can be properly understood', Winnicott did not publish any further work on smoking addiction.

If 'addiction can be stated in terms of regression to the early stage at which the transitional phenomena are unchallenged' (Winnicott, 1953, p. 97), and since smoking addiction is also a form of addiction, can we say that smoking addiction is also a regression to the early stage at which the transitional phenomena are unchallenged? And what is the role of cigarettes in this regressive behaviour? A PEP-Web search indicates that no paper has been published on the relationship between smoking addiction and regression or a regressed transitional object or transitional phenomena. The scarcity of papers published in the psychoanalytic field suggests that this is a highly original and under-researched area

If we follow Winnicott's theoretical framework, smoking addiction can be seen as a deprivation-triggered and artificially 'induced but unconsciously sought ego regression' (Wieder & Kaplan, 1969, p. 403) to a primitive state of blissful satiation and symbiotic dyad associated with the first year of life. The institution of the addictive state as transitional phenomena could be regarded as a desperate attempt by cigarette smokers to establish object contact at the expense of physiological decay, and eventually, death. As such, a cigarette can be seen as a regressed form of an infantile transitional object for smokers to cope with the infantile anxiety of separation and the loss of delusional omnipotence. However, the 'benefits' of cigarette usage are temporary because a cigarette is only a 'transitional' object; unlike Winnicott's healthy transitional object proper, which facilitates ego growth towards independence and real object relations, the absence of progressive adaptation or 'weaning' from the 'good-enough mother' in the addictive state suggests that cigarettes would continue to remain a necessity whenever the smokers needed to manage the anxiety of separation. The loss of delusional omnipotence in the face of deprivation, and a prolonged dependence on cigarettes would only render it a substitute for self-sustaining object relationships and prevent the acquisition and internalisation of essential regulatory functions, which are part of healthy ego development. Moreover, because the smokers continue to experience the 'benefits' of cigarettes as coming from the environment rather than from within themselves, this prolonged dependence on cigarettes would eventually lead to a state similar to the one experienced by marijuana addicts (Sugarman & Kurash 1982b, p. 535), i.e. 'confusion between inner and outer reality ... identity diffusion, disruption of the ego's synthetic function and inability to achieve higher levels of symbolisation'.

In a nutshell, according to Winnicott, transitional phenomena can be defined as:

> ... the intermediate area of experience, between the thumb and the teddy bear, between the oral erotism and true object-relationship, between primary creative activity and projection of what has already been introjected, between primary unawareness and indebtedness and the acknowledgement of indebtedness.
>
> (Winnicott, 1953, p. 89)

Transitional phenomena, transitional space, potential space, the intermediate area, and the third area are used interchangeably by Winnicott. This transitional space can only occur through trust and feelings of reliability towards the mother, and therefore towards other people and things. In health, all of us live in this transitional space throughout our entire lives. Our enjoyment in this transitional space will be pursued differently depending on which culture we are born into. This includes reading, playing football, dancing, etc.

There is a very close connection between the concept of transitional phenomena and a transitional object. In his 1953 paper, Winnicott provided a definition of a transitional object by stating that:

> ... out of all this (if we study any one infant) there may emerge some thing or some phenomenon – perhaps a bundle of wool or the corner of a blanket or eiderdown, or a word or tune, or a mannerism, which becomes vitally important to

the infant for use at the time of going to sleep, and is a defence against anxiety, especially anxiety of depressive type. Perhaps some soft object or type of object has been found and used by the infant, and this then becomes what I am calling a transitional object'

(Winnicott, 1953, p. 91)

A typical transitional object is a soft object within easy reach of the baby, usually part of a blanket, sheet, or other soft materials used by the mother for the baby. The transitional object serves oral erotism and in a certain way represents the mother. It is something that is 'created' by the baby between the age of four and twelve months. The important point here is that it must be perceived by the baby as its own creation and cannot be given to it by the mother directly, even though in reality it is indirectly given by the mother. The baby becomes attached to the transitional object, and it is demanded when the baby is about to go to sleep or at times of stress, when the object may be pressed against the baby's face and lips or sucked. When the baby is able to walk, it insists on taking it everywhere. The object retains the smell of the baby and the mother and it cannot be washed, and the baby would be in extreme distress if the object was misplaced, taken away, or lost.

Therefore, to Winnicott, a transitional object can be seen as a mother-substitute for the baby to deal with separation anxiety and the loss of omnipotence. The early stage of transitional phenomena and the presence of an infantile transitional object represent the existence of an intermediate space of reunion with the mother in the phantasy, and it is 'one of the bridges that make contact possible between the individual psyche and external reality' (Winnicott, 1955a, p. 218), and also 'a salient marker of an intermediate stage of transitional phenomena and functioning during which the baby is helped through good-enough maternal care to separate inner and outer worlds' (Abram, 2007, pp. 9–10).

Winnicott also suggests that a transitional object can be prolonged beyond early infancy when the infant is faced with deprivation:

Patterns set in infancy may persist into childhood, so that the original soft object continues to be absolutely necessary at bedtime or at time of loneliness or when a depressed mood threatens. In health, however, there is a gradual extension of range of interest, and eventually the extended range is maintained, even when depressive anxiety is near. A need for a specific object or a behaviour pattern that started at a very early date may reappear at a later age when deprivation threatens.

(Winnicott, 1953, p. 91)

We would argue that there is a high level of similarity between Winnicott's 'transitional object' and Menzies Lyth's 'pleasure food' (tobacco), as both objects are used as a powerful mother-substitute to ease off anxieties and depression, when confronted with deprivation reminiscent of their infantile anxieties. Winnicott's view on the reappearance of an infantile transitional object is also very similar to

Menzies Lyth's view when she categorised tobacco as a type of 'pleasure food' similar to ice cream, and that 'pleasure foods' (tobacco) are used as a powerful mother-substitute (towards whom the infant has ambivalent feelings), in order to ease anxiety and depression when an individual is confronted with deprivation reminiscent of his infantile anxieties.

> Ice cream belongs to a group of products which may be described as pleasure foods ... Closely associated, though not actually eaten or drunk, are tobacco and chewing gym. These products are related to certain psychological and social factors and characteristic of them is their ability to gratify oral desires and, like the breast with the infant, change depression and anxiety into pleasure... This kind of oral gratification serves, then as a method of alleviating current anxieties and depression which are in part the derivatives of the infantile anxiety and depression connected with the actual loss of the breast. Compensation for this loss is sought in the consumption of substitute objects, the pleasure foods. Thus the need for them becomes particularly great when contemporary difficulties awaken again the residues of the earlier situations which to a greater or lesser extent exist in anyone.
>
> (Menzies Lyth, 1989, pp. 71–72)

In consultation with Jan Abram and Lesley Caldwell (Personal communications), the idea around the reappearance of an infantile transitional object in adulthood in a concrete form, such as a cigarette, seems to be paradoxical and problematic. The reason is that theoretically speaking, a transitional object belongs to the infantile period, and that it should have already been 'relegated to limbo' in adulthood (Winnicott, 1953, p. 91). Having said that, if we approach the idea from Winnicott's notion of 'regression' and his view that 'addiction can be stated in terms of regression to the earliest stage at which the transitional phenomena are unchallenged' (1953, p. 97), then the reappearance of an infantile transitional object in the form of a concrete object, that is, a cigarette, becomes theoretically possible.

To summarise, what we have established from the above are:

1. Addiction can be seen as a regression to the infantile transitional phenomena.
2. A transitional object is a salient marker of the transitional phenomena, which usually appears at the age of four to twelve months.
3. A transitional object can be prolonged beyond early infancy and reappear in later life when deprivation threatens.

Since this is a book looking at the value of Winnicott's transitional object as a concept to understand smoking addiction, the perspectives of Freud's sexual phantasies and Klein's introjection (inhaling) of internal objects are beyond the scope of this book.

Part IV

Which research approach has the power to access the unconscious?

If a cigarette is a regressed form of infantile 'transitional object' that prolongs into adulthood, then there must be a powerful force in the unconscious that strengthens addiction to smoking. Anything 'infantile' should have been repressed, and the location of the 'transitional object' is in-between the internal and the external world, which means it is neither from within nor from without. Therefore, to shed light on how a cigarette acts like a regressed form of infantile 'transitional object', we need a method of enquiry that has the power to tap into the repressed materials and infer the unconscious. The Free Association Narrative Interview (Hollway & Jefferson, 2013) method was chosen as the primary data collection method in view of its power to access the unconscious and embedded emotional experiences through eliciting free associations from respondents.

We will first describe the limitations of quantitative survey-based research in providing contextual meanings to the data, and the failure of traditional qualitative interview-based research to address this, including grounded theory, interpretative phenomenological analysis, and discourse analysis. We will then describe how the narrative and psychoanalytic clinical case-study approach can overcome the limitations identified in traditional quantitative and qualitative research. We will explain how the Free Association Narrative Interview through the incorporation of the psychoanalytic concepts of the unconscious defence against anxiety, 'free association', transference and countertransference, into the narrative interview method, can provide a much more detailed picture and richer insight for emotionally-charged and identity-based issues. In conclusion, we will propose a research approach based on the Free Association Narrative Interview method.

Key sections

- Quantitative survey-based research?
- Qualitative interview-based research?
- The narrative interviewing approach?
- The Free Association Narrative Interview (FANI) method!
- What does our research approach look like?

DOI: 10.4324/9781003329077-13

Chapter 9

Quantitative survey-based research?

Garbage in, garbage out

Quantitative survey-based research requires all collected data to be reduced to numerical values in order to facilitate a statistical analysis, therefore quantitative research is effective in describing numbers and counts of easily measurable factors generated by closed-ended questions, such as the percentage of smokers in a population or age distribution and gender split of smokers. However, it fails to answer the 'what does this mean?' and 'why is that?' questions on more complex and unquantifiable factors, such as why some people smoke but some do not, given the similar level of exposure to tobacco marketing campaign and peer group influence.

With its heavy reliance on quantifying and coding isolated responses on a Likert scale, and subsequent artificial re-aggregation into different demographic subgroups, quantitative survey-based research tends to group everything into a single artificial entity, measured through one hypothetical closed question. It de-contextualises the respondent's answers because it fails to take into consideration the socio-cultural meaning of these responses. Given these limitations, the resultant artificial aggregations would end up having no direct representation in the real world.

DOI: 10.4324/9781003329077-14

Chapter 10

Qualitative interview-based research?

Issues with transparency of account, transparency of self, and transparency of others

In response to the weaknesses of quantitative survey-based research, qualitative interview-based research, with its more in-depth, semi-structured, face-to-face interview approach, attempts to give voice to the respondents and find out more about the contextual meanings of their experiences. Contrary to quantitative survey-based research, qualitative interview-based research involves collecting data in the form of verbal reports and the analysis is textual instead of statistical. It relies heavily on the interpretation of the collected text and, as such, there is a theoretical underpinning of the value of language as a fundamental communication tool between human beings.

In the following sections, we will describe in detail the theoretical underpinnings, as well as the strengths, of three major qualitative data analysis approaches, including grounded theory, interpretative phenomenological analysis, and discourse analysis, followed by an overall evaluation of these three analytic approaches.

Grounded theory

Grounded theory is a technique of analysis developed by Barney Glaser and Anselm Strauss (1967) aiming at developing theoretical constructs and empirical knowledge from analysing and interpreting qualitative data. It is a comparative and interactive method that encapsulates a set of systematic guidelines for collecting, synthesising, analysing, and conceptualising qualitative data to build inductive theories, which can be later verified through other traditional quantitative research methodologies, so the resultant theoretical theories are directly 'grounded' in the collected data, that is, a bottom-up approach. Because of this characteristic, ground theory excels in theory revisions, as well as providing a useful strategy for researchers to review and reformulate their research methods (Corbin & Strauss, 2008).

Interpretative Phenomenological Analysis (IPA)

IPA is a qualitative research methodology inspired by Husserlian phenomenology. It examines how people make sense of major life experiences through

DOI: 10.4324/9781003329077-15

semi-structured interviews and interpretation by the researcher. IPA researchers see these more significant life experiences as comprising a range of fragments of life that are separated in time but linked with a common meaning and theme, and the objective of the interviews is to encourage the respondents' recall of these disconnected fragments in order to rebuild their connections and discover the hidden common meanings and themes. The core strength of IPA lies in its ability to shed light on the human predicament and on how human beings engage with the world. However, it is also prone to the possibility of errors in memory or intentional deceits from the respondents in their retrospective accounts; moreover, since the entire data analysis relies solely on the interpretation provided by the researchers, it is highly subjective and thus results in a lack of totally neutral access to the subject matter being researched (Smith, 2008; Smith et al., 2009).

Discourse analysis

Instead of seeing language as a set of objective and distinctive signs to describe internal states and external reality, discourse analysts argue that language should be regarded as productive and constructive in nature, and that it plays a key role in constructing social reality for individuals to achieve personal and social objectives. This 'turning to language' movement that began in the 1980s, resulted in a shift of the qualitative research inquiry's focus from individuals and their intentions to language and its productive and constructive potential. Discourse analysts focus on going beyond the manifest content of the text to trace its action orientation and internal organisation within a specific social context in order to uncover the underlying meaning and implications of the text. It can be seen as a special approach in reading a text, underpinned by the fundamental assumption of language as productive and performative in nature. All talk and text are treated as social action and this orientation directs the analytic work of discourse analysis (Smith, 2008).

The major problem with traditional qualitative research, including the three major qualitative analysis methodologies described here, is that they assume that words mean the same thing to both researchers and respondents, and there is a commonly agreed shared meaning attached to words used in interviews, that is, the meanings of the questions asked by the researchers are assumed to be the same as the meanings that are understood by the respondents, and vice versa with regard to the answers provided by the respondents. This assumption of shared meanings between researchers and respondents is still based on the positivist view of a rational unitary respondent, who carries the same assumptions as those of the quantitative researchers (Hollway & Jefferson, 2013). Traditional qualitative research also suffers from the highly questionable assumptions that respondents are knowledgeable about their actions and feelings, and they are willing and able to recount them to a stranger (researcher).

Due to the limitations of the above methodologies, a different research approach to access respondents' unconscious materials and structure is required to shed light on our enquiry.

Chapter 11

The narrative interviewing approach?

Tell me whatever that comes to your mind

As opposed to the traditional qualitative interview approach which follows a structured or semi-structured interviewing agenda in which the researchers set the agenda and are in full control of the information produced throughout the interview, in the narrative interviewing approach, the researchers take a more passive role by only selecting the theme, topics and sequence of the interview.

It follows that the researcher's role in the narrative approach is to be a good listener and the respondent's role is to be a story-teller. The agenda is open to development and change by the respondents, and any attempt to impose a traditional question-and-answer interviewing approach would only interrupt the flow and suppress the respondents' stories (Bauer, 1996; Jovchelovitch & Bauer, 2000). The biographical-interpretative method (Schütze, 1992a, 1992b; Rosenthal, 1993) belongs to the narrative interview tradition. Its main theoretical principle is the notion that there exists a 'gestalt', a meaning-frame, a holistic form or a whole that is greater than the sum of its parts, governing each person's life. The researchers are responsible for assisting the respondents to provide a more intact life story, and hence facilitate the emergence of 'gestalt'. In this approach, the researcher should not provide interpretations, judgements, impose their own meaning-frame, or follow a pre-determined interview agenda that only addresses the researcher's interests, because to do so would destroy the 'gestalt' or the respondent's meaning.

DOI: 10.4324/9781003329077-16

Chapter 12

The Free Association Narrative Interview (FANI) method!

A powerful tool to unearth the anxieties of the 'defended subject'

The Free Association Narrative Interview (FANI) method was first developed by Wendy Hollway and Tony Jefferson on the publication of the first edition of their ground-breaking book *Doing qualitative research differently: a psychosocial approach*. It is a qualitative research method for the production and analysis of face-to-face interview data that is grounded on the narrative approach and guided by the psychoanalytic principles of 'free association'. This method uses open-ended questions to elicit narratives that are linked to specific events from respondents. Unlike intellectualised and generalised de-contextualised accounts that are emotionally drained, the stories elicited from respondents are highly charged with emotional connotations. According to the principle of 'free association', the emotional significance of respondent accounts is usually contained in the links, arranged in a certain sequence, between the seemingly inconsistent fragments of elicited narratives, rather than their rational content. In view of the strengths of the FANI method compared to the traditional qualitative research method in accessing the unconscious and embodied emotional experiences through eliciting free associations from the participants, it will be chosen as the primary data collection method to explore the relationship between smokers and cigarettes, and how that relationship resembles the infantile transitional object that extends into adulthood in a regressed form.

The FANI method is grounded on the key principles of psychoanalytic theories. Its data collection method is driven by 'free association' and its data analysis is based on interpretation. There are a few key assumptions that differentiate the FANI method from a conventional qualitative research approach. This includes the notion of the 'defended subject' and the need to view the respondents as psychosocial instead of rational unitary subjects. Emphasis is placed on the use of the researcher's subjectivity as an instrument of knowing, and the need to respect the 'gestalt' of respondents' accounts (Hollway & Jefferson, 2013).

DOI: 10.4324/9781003329077-17

Key ideas

- Yes, you are a 'defended subject'
- Trust your instincts and feelings
- Look at the big picture
- What? We don't have a control group?
- Can we trust the results?
- What ethical responsibilities do we have towards the respondents?

Yes, you are a 'defended subject'

According to the Kleinian notion of unconscious defence against anxiety, the infant's early experience is dominated by acute anxiety in the face of complete dependency, and polarised emotions of 'good' when it is fed and 'bad' when it is hungry. Unable to recognise a whole object, the infant mentally splits between all good experiences, associated with a 'good' part-object that is loved, and all bad experiences, associated with a 'bad' part-object that is frantically attacked. These two part-objects are kept mentally separated for the defensive purpose to protect the 'good' from the 'bad'. Klein called this the 'paranoid-schizoid position' and this position is filled with destructive impulses.

As the infant's ego becomes more developed and integrated, it is capable of realising that both the loved 'good' and the hated 'bad' part-objects actually belong to the same whole object, and a sense of ambivalence develops towards the whole object as the mother begins to be seen as capable of both 'good' and 'bad'. This is when love and hate, external reality and internal phantasy, co-exist in the infant's mind. The infant begins to acknowledge its own dependency and helplessness towards the mother and starts to feel anxious about its previous aggressive impulses, fearing that it may have destroyed the same mother that it loves. This characterises the Kleinian 'depressive position' and is replete with depressive anxiety and guilt feelings.

According to Klein, the self is continuously shaped by unconscious defences against anxiety since birth. The self is not a single unit with clear boundaries separating it from the external world; these unconscious defences against anxieties are inter-subjective and occur in relation to the external objects, for example, splitting is achieved through the projection of a 'bad' internal object and the introjection of a 'good' external object. Anxiety is inherent in the human condition, and people constantly move between the 'paranoid-schizoid position' and the 'depressive position' when faced with deprivations in the threatening world, depending on the perceived level of threat and the level of development of the ego, even though different people do have a tendency to respond with one or the other position.

The ideas of unconscious anxieties and the 'defended subject' suggest that both quantitative and qualitative research traditions view the research respondents as rationally driven and socially constructed unitary individuals and this is problematic. The internal world of the respondents should not be viewed simply as a reflection or a rational interpretation of the external world; rather it needs to be understood through the lens of their unconscious anxieties and defences, which operate at an unconscious level exerting a significant influence on their lives, their relations with others, and their everyday actions. These unconscious defences determine how the respondents experience their external world, or how they interpret events and extract meanings in the research context.

Trust your instincts and feelings

The FANI method assumes that all research respondents are meaning-seeking and anxious defended subjects who may not share the same meaning-frame as the researchers or other respondents, and they are also invested in particular 'positions' as a defence mechanism for ego protection purposes. As such, they may not know the reasons behind their feelings and behaviours, and they are unconsciously motivated to disguise the meanings of at least part of their feelings and behaviours.

The researchers, at the same time, share many similarities with the respondents. They are also anxious and defended individuals who are subject to projections and introjections of emotions and feelings coming from the respondents in the research context. This means that the impressions that the research pair gain from each other should not be seen as deriving from a real and objective relationship; instead, they are coloured by unconscious phantasies derived from significant relationships in the past, accessible only through feelings, not rational understanding and conscious awareness. As such, the researcher is encouraged to make use of their emotional responses to the interview in data analysis, as they are of value in understanding the dynamics of the research relationship, which is aided by keeping a record of detailed, reflexive field notes. Given the above theoretical starting point, all data in the research context is co-produced by the research pair, in which unconscious intersubjective dynamics, transference and countertransference are in full operation.

Hollway and Jefferson's notion of the 'defended subject' is both psychic and social. It is psychic because its development is driven by a unique biography of anxiety-provoking life events that have been unconsciously defended against. It is also social because of its intimate relationship with external events and objects, and the associated interpretations and experiences of these external entities. It is this psychosocial nature of the anxious and defended subjects that provides additional depth and insight into the 'what', 'how', and 'who' of the research results.

For instance, as reported by Hollway and Jefferson (1997) in their 'fear of crime' study, demographic and geographic clustering failed to account for the differences in the respondents' perceived risk of crime. However, when positing the respondents as biographically unique 'defended subjects' investing in specific discourses and 'positions' that shielded them against unconscious anxieties, a more complete picture emerged, and an understanding of differences between respondents that were not explainable by demographic and geographic clustering was obtained. Therefore, identical demographic and geographic profiles should not be the basis for generalising research findings because they could be achieved as a result of very different respondent biographies. In order to obtain the full picture, any attempt at generalisation must be based on a combination of biographic, demographic and geographic factors.

Look at the big picture

When analysing narrative data using the FANI method, it is important not to interpret the respondents' accounts taken at face value, since they are likely to be driven by the respondents' post-rationalisation in order to appear consistent and coherent. In order to understand the meaning of narrated stories and to make sense of the apparent inconsistencies, it is important to first take a broader look at the whole of the evidence through an understanding of the entire transcript materials. This is very different from the 'code and retrieve' data analysis system adopted by the traditional qualitative researcher, which would lead to a fragmentation and decontextualisation of the information. Second, it is important to utilise the theory of the 'defended subject' in order to understand the respondents' investment in a particular discourse, as a result of the activation of an unconscious defence mechanism against anxieties. Finally, researchers using this method are encouraged to leverage on their reflexivity by investing time and effort in recording notes containing their subjective experiences and feelings immediately after each interview. When used properly, reflexivity may help to reinforce a theoretical conviction or alert the researchers to a potential misreading of the information. With the above three principles in mind, together with information gathered from respondent's narrated stories through 'free associations', unconscious inter-subjective dynamics involving transference and countertransference, and the application of psychoanalytic knowledge, the next step is for the researchers to begin creating links to re-join the disconnected elements from the data and provide form to the respondents' account.

What? We don't have a control group?

According to Hinshelwood (2013), research in psychoanalysis can be broadly divided into two types. The first type is outcome research of clinical trials with the objective of measuring the effectiveness of psychoanalytic treatments. This type of research is mostly quantitative, and it arises as a result of financial pressures within healthcare institutions, hence the need to justify the effectiveness of psychoanalytic treatment versus other types of treatment. The second type is conceptual research about basic theoretical ideas in psychoanalysis which precedes clinical work, similar to the Menninger Psychotherapy Research Project pioneered by Wallerstein between 1954 and 1982. This is also the type of research that Freud used to derive psychoanalytic knowledge based on the single-case study, rather than from massed and aggregated samples of large numbers of subjects. In fact, the majority of psychoanalytic knowledge has come from clinical cases based on a single-case study approach without a control group.

The single-case study research tradition used by Freud was also advocated by Winnicott, as seen in the talks given to pupils at St Paul's School in London, and to students of psychology and social work at the London School of Economics:

Psychology simply means the study of human nature, and that it is a science, just as physics, physiology, and biology are sciences.

(Winnicott, 1945, p. 381)

True intuition can reach to a whole truth in a flash (just as faulty intuition can reach to error), whereas in a science the whole truth is never reached. What is important in science is a construction of a satisfactory road towards the truth … If, in a subject that is being approached through the scientific method, there is a gap in our knowledge, we just record it as a gap in knowledge, a stimulus to research, but the intuitive person's gaps are unknown quantities with somewhat terrifying potential … The scientific approach to the phenomena of human nature enables us to be ignorant without being frightened, and without, therefore, having to invent all sorts of weird theories to explain away the gaps in knowledge.

(Winnicott, 1945, p. 383)

No wonder it is difficult to learn about psychology. What is the answer? One thing is to go slow. Another is to get relief from the fact that some of what is taught is bound to be wrong, although psychology can teach a good deal about human nature that is true as far as it goes.

(Winnicott, 1950, p. 426)

In the rapidly changing context of healthcare requiring a systematised method of testing theories, there has been an increasing emphasis on an evidence-based approach for outcome research in psychoanalysis. The contested nature of the current debates within psychoanalysis around themes of quantitative versus qualitative research can be seen in the debate between Kernberg and Perron published in the *International Journal of Psychoanalysis* in 2006 (Scott, 2018).

As Scott (2018) suggests, despite differences between the inductive tradition of qualitative research and deductive reasoning and testing required for quantitative research, they should not be regarded as mutually exclusive. This can be seen in the increasing number of mixed-methods research approaches that use elements of both qualitative and quantitative approaches. One example is the Tavistock Adult Depression Study conducted between 2002 and 2013, which used a combination of a pragmatic, randomised controlled trial to compare the treatment effectiveness of a group of patients who received 18 months of weekly psychoanalytic psychotherapy, versus a control group who received other forms of treatment approved by NICE and administered by their General Practitioner. This outcome trial was completed by a two-year follow-up after treatment completion using clinical research and qualitative research methodology (The Tavistock and Portman NHS Foundation Trust, 2018).

However, it is also possible to conduct clinical research in a classically Freudian tradition, as demonstrated by Hinshelwood's cogent logical model to test psychoanalytic theories clinically (2013). As suggested by Hinshelwood, it is a model that enables us to:

> forget the suspicion of single-case studies which can prove to be more definitive than large sample testing, given the right conditions;
>
> acknowledge the subjectivity of the field of investigation without being apologetic about it, since it is the unique contribution of psychoanalysis;
>
> retain causality and the possibility of prediction, while simultaneously keeping the subjective meaning and narrative to the fore; and
>
> face the challenge of developing facts that are not biased to one or another psychoanalytic school.
>
> (Hinshelwood, 2013, pp. 33–34)

In the long run, psychoanalysis as a unique body of knowledge centred around understanding a subjective human experience can benefit from an evidence-based approach to research. A two-pronged strategy for research design in psychoanalysis can help our engagement with dialogue outside the psychoanalytic community, through the use of an outward-facing quantitative approach and at the same time, we can also remain loyal to the tradition of conceptual research based on inductive reasoning through an inward-facing approach advocated by Freud, and further developed by Hinshelwood (2013).

Can we trust the results?

A positivist epistemology requires that all knowledge must be directly linked to observable events, with objectivity and reliability as the definitive criteria (Hollway and Jefferson, 2013). In relation to the principle of objectivity, with its heavy reliance on intuition, emotion, feelings, researcher subjectivity, inter-subjectivity of the research pair, and the use of unconscious dynamics as a technique to derive insight, it is commonly acknowledged in the psychoanalytic field that psychoanalytic interpretation is an art, not a science, thus the principle of objectivity is beyond the scope of the psychoanalytic principle and the FANI method. In the face of criticism and doubt on the validity of the knowledge generated by psychoanalysis, one useful defence is the integrity of the methodology and persuasiveness of the clinical evidence contained in the narratives and interpretations of the research data.

With regard to the second principle of reliability, which requires consistency, stability, and repeatability of results, it is an invalid principle for psychoanalysis and the FANI method because it assumes that meanings can be controlled in every single application of a question. In psychoanalysis, situations and respondents for each psychoanalytic encounter will never be the same, and meanings are unique to the respondents and the relational encounters. Therefore, the results generated by the FANI method should be regarded as reliable, as long as the interpretations are grounded in sound theoretical principles, the results are firmly empirical with supporting evidence, and similar interpretations can be obtained by different researchers.

What ethical responsibilities do we have towards the respondents?

As stipulated in the ethical principles published by the British Psychological Society (2021), ethical issues in social science research primarily concern ensuring the welfare and interests of research respondents and require the researcher to report his findings truthfully and accurately. When translated into research practice, these ethical standards mean an informed consent must be obtained from the respondents, no harm must be inflicted, and all information obtained must be treated in strict confidence to ensure the anonymity of the respondents.

However, Hollway and Jefferson (2013) point out that ethical principles may not be applicable for researching psychosocial subjects in the FANI method due to a number of reasons. First, due to the nature of the method, where there is no pre-determined list interview questions, it is the respondents who are in control of what and how the narrated stories are told in the interview. Hence, it is not possible to predict how each respondent would experience the interview encounter, and it is also impossible to brief respondents in advance accordingly in a meaningful way. Second, while it is against ethical practice for researchers to inflict harm on the respondents, a key question is whether it is necessarily harmful for the respondents to experience distress in the interview, given the known therapeutic effect of engaging in discussion of disturbing events within a safe and controlled psychoanalytic environment. In the realm of psychoanalysis, unconscious defence protects the respondent against the painful 'truth', therefore it follows that a 'truthful' analysis may indeed inflict distress and anxiety on the respondents, but such distress and anxiety should not be automatically linked to 'harm'.

Given the co-creative nature of the FANI method, both researchers and respondents are active co-participants in the data produced, and what is said and revealed in the interview can only be known during, and not before, the interview. Therefore, the fundamental criterion to determine the ethical standard for the FANI method should not be informed consent, but rather on the issue of avoiding harm, which in turns relies on the researchers' responsibility for creating a safe interviewing environment based on honesty, sympathy, and respect. Finally, with regard to the ethical requirement to ensure the anonymity of respondents, the likelihood of concealing the respondents' identities in published biographical research is extremely difficult without significantly distorting the original data, especially for those having a certain distinctive combination of attributes. Furthermore, the use of data from members of the same family, neighbourhood, or organisation poses further challenges to the requirements of absolute confidentiality. The only way to ensure anonymity is to refrain from publication of case studies, but that would be against the wider interest of making the knowledge publicly available. As such, it is imperative for the researchers to ensure that any potential objections on the publication of the results, alternative interpretations of the data, and views of the respondents have been thoroughly examined and considered in the final research report, and that no greater level of harm than might be predicted is inflicted on the respondents, compared to the level they have already been exposed to.

In view of the limitations of the current ethical principles in researching psychosocial subjects, Hollway and Jefferson (2013) propose a more suitable set of ethical principles that is built around the values of honesty, sympathy and respect. To be specific, honesty means approaching the collected data in the spirit of inquiry instead of advocacy, leveraging on a sound theoretical framework that is justified, and making only interpretations that can be supported by solid evidence. Sympathy refers to the researchers' capacity to take the perspective of the respondents, sharing their feelings and emotions. The ethical principle of respect refers to the notion of carefully observing the research subjects with complete attention to ensure that there is a realistic appraisal that is independent of our own defences, as well as analysing the collected data using our theoretical, empirical, and experiential knowledges in order to observe what might be too painful for the client to notice.

Chapter 13

What does our research approach look like?

In view of the strengths of the Free Association Narrative Interview (FANI) method (Hollway & Jefferson, 2013), compared to the traditional qualitative research method, in accessing the unconscious and embodied emotional experiences through eliciting free associations from participants, we conducted interviews with smokers using the primary data collection method in order to explore the relationship between smokers and cigarettes, and observe how it resembles the infantile transitional object that extends into adulthood in a regressed form. However, contrary to traditional qualitative research, the role of the researcher in the FANI method is to be an attentive listener, and the respondents assume the role of storytellers who recount their life stories.

Key ideas

- Two interviews, one week apart
- Five open narrative questions
- Who are the respondents?
- How many respondents do we have?
- How do we make sense of the data?

Two interviews, one week apart

Using the FANI approach, a total of two, one-hour interviews, one to two weeks apart, with each participant were completed. Consent forms on research participation, and voice and video recordings for each interview were also obtained with the agreement of all eight respondents. The first interview was intented to establish a preliminary reading of the elicited narratives, to critically interrogate what was said, and to pick up any contradictions and inconsistencies, defensive avoidances, and changes of tone. The purpose of the second interview was for the researcher to seek further evidence and clarifications from the respondents in order to confirm provisional hypotheses and analyses.

DOI: 10.1324/9781003329077-18

The one- to two-week gap between the two interviews also allowed for time for the researcher to reflect on what was said in the first interview, which is critical in the FANI method, as it involves using the researcher's subjectivity as an instrument of knowing, and without reflection it would be difficult to correctly grasp emotional factors and transform them into useful insight.

Five open narrative questions

In consultation with Professor Wendy Hollway, the co-developer of the FANI method, it was found that there is value in asking some fairly open, but specific, narrative questions (personal communications). Responses to these might have significant bearing on our main research questions. Interview questions were open-ended and intentionally designed to elicit experience-near narratives that require psychological depth from the participants, and at the same time allowed for free associations to emerge, and minimised the occurrences of opinion-based generalisation and post-rationalisation. The objective was to uncover the emotional footings of the experiences recounted by participants in the research interviews.

Narrative questions for the first interview:

1. Can you tell me about a recent happy moment in your life and how you felt about it?
2. Can you tell me about a recent distressing moment in your life and how you coped with it?
3. I am interested in smokers' embodied experience of cigarettes. Can you tell me how it felt yesterday to smoke your favourite cigarette of the day?
4. Can you tell me the most disappointing cigarette that you remember smoking recently?
5. Can you tell me the ideal cigarette that you remember smoking recently?

Narrative questions for the second interview

In the first interview we established a preliminary reading based on critical interrogation of what was said, and we identified inconsistences, contradictions, avoidances, hesitations, and changes in emotional tone. Following that stage, we reviewed and reflected on the recordings of the first interview. In the second interview, which was conducted one to two weeks later, we followed up on themes and issues that appeared to suggest tensions. The second interview also gave us the opportunity to acquire further evidence in order to test the hunches and provisional hypotheses established in the first interview.

Who are the respondents?

In order to minimise the social factors contributing to smoking addiction, including sociocultural factors such as the awareness of public health campaigns, the level of exposure to the risk of smoking, and generational factors, we narrowed the recruitment criteria to include only students aged between 18 to 24, who were studying in tertiary institutions in Hong Kong, and whose parents were non-smokers.

The above criteria were chosen because, first, tobacco advertising on electronic media was banned in Hong Kong on 1 December 1990. This date, many years before our participants were born, would have limited their exposure to the most powerful form of above-the-line tobacco advertising, therefore minimising sociocultural factors affecting smoking addiction as far as possible. Second, undergraduate students are assumed to have a better understanding than the general public of the risks of smoking cigarettes. Third, by choosing participants whose parents are non-smokers, a generational influence on smoking may also be minimised.

How many respondents do we have?

In line with the principles of the FANI method, the sample size of this research was not meant to correspond to the requirements of statistical generalisability. In order to enable extrapolations of concepts and potential explanations from qualitative case data and, to some extent, identifying patterning amongst single cases, we aimed to maximise the variation amongst the respondents within the above sampling frame. Within the limitations of a sample size that permits sufficient depth, depth trumps breadth as a criterion in this research, and the aim was to maximise variation amongst participants. The criteria for dimensions of variations in order to optimise the strength of our sample include the gender of the participants, whether they have siblings or not, and whether they were raised by both parents or a single parent.

A total of eight smokers from tertiary institutions in Hong Kong were recruited through Field and Tab Research Services Limited to reflect the above sample variations. This was to ensure that we gathered sufficiently rich data in order to generate suggestive ideas to take forward from hypothesis substantiation to a theoretical concept development. The respondents were then invited by Field and Tab Research Services Limited to a main meeting room at their office for the interviews. Each respondent was given a project information sheet that contained information related to the objectives, duration, and frequency of the interviews. They were informed that all the interviews would be video recorded and transcribed for research analysis purposes. They were reassured of anonymity and confidentiality, and that they could withdraw at any time without giving any reasons for doing so. All of the respondents were required to sign a consent form upon agreement to take part in the interviews.

For the profiles of the eight recruited and interviewed respondents, see Table 13.1.

Table 13.1 Profile of the respondents

Profile of respondents						
Age range		18–24 (students in tertiary institutions in Hong Kong)				
Gender		4 Male		4 Female		
Parents' smoking status		All non-smokers				
Parents' marital status		4 Married		4 Divorced		

Name (anonymised)	Gender	Age	Regularly smoked cigarette brand	Average daily consumption (no. of sticks)	Parents' marital status	Sibling
Hank	Male	19	Marlboro Medium Red	20	Married	1 brother
Anthony	Male	21	Lamborghini	10	Married	1 brother
Holly	Female	20	Marlboro Ice Blast	10	Married	Single child
Anita	Female	21	Mild Seven	5	Married	Single child
Cooper	Female	20	Marlboro Blue Ice	10	Divorced	1 sister
Emerald	Female	23	Pianissimo	8	Divorced	1 sister
Abyss	Male	21	Marlboro Black	20	Divorced	Single child
Samuel	Male	21	Marlboro Double Capsule	10	Divorced	Single child

How do we make sense of the data?

In order to answer the research question, 'To what extent can a cigarette be regarded as a regressed form of infantile transitional object that prolongs into adulthood?', we used three levels of analysis to examine the collected interview data. First, we used the FANI method in order to identify the 'defended smoking moments' as manifested in the interviews. This was followed by comparing themes extracted from the data with the 'smoking moments' from tobacco industry research, in order to identify the highly personal and regressive smoking moments out of the six personal moments, that is, 'pass the time', 'me time', 'self-reward', 'relax', 'focus/problem solver', and 'boost/start up' moments (please refer to the literature review for a more detailed description of the 'smoking moments' research conducted by the tobacco industry, pp. 20–26). Finally, we used Winnicott's seven criteria of transitional objects (1953) to locate specific instances of the occurrence of the regressed transitional object in the interviews:

1. The infant assumes rights over the object …
2. The object is affectionately cuddled as well as excitedly loved and mutilated.
3. It must never be changed, unless changed by the infant.
4. It must survive instinctual loving, and also hating …

5. Yet it must seem to the infant to give warmth, or to move, or to have texture, or to do something that seems to show it has vitality or reality of its own.

6. It comes from without from our point of view, but not so from the point of view of the baby. Neither does it come from within ...

7. Its fate is to be gradually allowed to be decathected, so that in the course of years it becomes not so much forgotten as relegated to limbo ...

(Winnicott, 1953, p. 91)

Part V

The shadow of the transitional object fell upon the cigarette

Each of the eight respondents have their own very unusual and unique story. This very private information was revealed to the researcher despite the limited number of interview sessions available and limited duration of each interview as per the FANI research set up, that is, two, one-hour interviews, one to two weeks apart for each respondent, indicating the power of letting respondents control the flow of their narratives, and getting the researcher to take a back seat.

The Free Association Narrative Interview (FANI) method is able to evoke rich narratives of the emotionally charged smoking moments, as well as providing in-depth insights on what smoking and cigarettes really mean to smokers and the relationship between them. The wealth and depth of information revealed by the FANI method is extremely powerful compared to commercial qualitative research, which the researcher has been exposed to in the past 30 years of her marketing career in the tobacco industry,

This part is divided into three chapters.

Key sections

- Our respondents – what are their stories?
- Spotting the 'regressive' smoking moments
- The resemblance of a cigarette to the transitional object

In Chapter 14, a pen portrait depicting the unique personal story of each respondent based on the field notes written by the researcher immediately after each interview is provided. Each pen portrait covers the demographic information of the respondents, their family and school lives, how they started smoking, and their relationship with cigarettes. Since this is a book about smoking addiction, a more detailed elaboration on the respondents' relationship with smoking will also be included in the pen portraits.

In Chapter 15, in order to provide a more systematic description of the respondents' relationship with cigarettes, a tobacco industry's commercial research

DOI: 10.4324/9781003329077-19

(see Part I, Chapter 2, 'What do the tobacco boys think' for details of the research) has been used to provide a framework to summarise how cigarettes are used by the respondents across different smoking moments; out of the eight smoking moments, the 'time out' and 'discharge' personal smoking moments emerged consistently across all the eight respondents' verbatims – compared to the other smoking moments, these are the more 'regressive' smoking moments that involve a fluid sort of regression and movement between internal and external realities triggered by stressful feelings.

In Chapter 16, we will take a closer look at how the respondents' smoking experience and their relationship with cigarettes resembles the seven qualities of transitional object outlined by Winnicott (1953). It was found that two of these qualities: the transitional object being perceived to have a life of its own, and its location as in between the inner and outer reality, manifested consistently in all the interviews of the eight respondents. Relevant snippets of the respondents' verbatim statements describing the emotionally charged smoking moments that resemble the qualities of the transitional object are provided.

Chapter 14

Our respondents – what are their stories?

Hank: a teenager who survived a craniotomy two months after birth due to infant meningitis

Hank is a 19-year-old, Year 1 university student in Hong Kong. Hank comes from a middle-class family and has a brother who is one year younger than him. His father is a businessman, but strangely enough, Hank does not know what kind of business his father has. The only thing he remembers is that his father was always out of town when he was a child, and sometimes his mother also travelled with his father, so he and his brother always ended up ordering take-outs for dinner. Hank's mother used to be a manager at a cosmetic store, but she decided to resign her position and become a full-time housewife when Hank sustained a fever and was diagnosed with acute meningitis two months after birth. Hank was admitted to hospital and endured a major operation to relieve the pressure on the brain. Hank was told by his mother that he underwent a craniotomy using a fragment of the chest bone of his cousin who was 15 months old. These major surgeries resulted in prolonged hospitalisation and separation from his mother for months immediately after his birth. This also explains why his mother was willing to give up her career in order to become a full-time housewife and look after Hank from that incident onwards.

Hank was expelled from a renowned elite high school in Hong Kong when he was in 16 years old due to truancy. He did not like his school, feeling suffocated and caged by the strict rules and regulations. He also did not like any of his class-mates there and preferred to hang out with another group of friends that he met on Facebook. Many of them were from elite boys schools and all of them were smokers. That was also the time when Hank started smoking – five years ago, when he was 14 years old, out of peer influence and curiosity. Hank said he felt relieved and happy after being expelled, he stopped studying for an entire year and instead waited for his friends outside their schools to go to game arcades, snooker clubs, and smoke together after school. However, after a while, with the influence of his girlfriend, he decided that he needed to go back to school in order to have a better future. Therefore, he went to Australia for six months, but he didn't like it, so he came back to Hong Kong and entered an international high school. Later on, he was finally admitted to a university in Hong Kong.

DOI: 10.4324/9781003329077-20

For Hank, smoking is an enjoyment, not something to be done in a hurry. He chooses high tar, full flavour cigarettes, as he enjoys the kick and the sensation, and he will not switch to low tar cigarettes or compromise on taste and satisfaction. He smoked his favourite cigarette of the day at noon on the day of our interview, alone, sitting outside his school and eating his lunch. The sensation of the sun washing over his whole body while he was smoking was so comforting, and the sensation of euphoria could not be expressed in words. Hank spoke of the most difficult and saddest moment of his life when he found out that his girlfriend had cheated on him with his best friend a year ago. This happened during his open exam time, when he only had his cigarettes and guitar to console him. Hank also likes to bite the cigarette filter, as he feels that he can draw more smoke into his lungs while smoking, so the front ends of his cigarettes are always soaking wet and have deep tooth marks all over them by the time he has finished smoking.

Hank uses cigarettes mainly for the 'time out' moments: he spoke about his most recent ideal cigarette at the harbour front during lunchtime, when he felt very comfortable and free from all the unhappiness while he was enjoying his smoke. Smoking a cigarette is like swallowing an 'air' of anger to him, and when this 'air' of anger is swallowed, it then disappears completely. Besides, he also mentioned a few times in the interviews that smoking is a wonderful feeling, and it allows him a short period of isolation from the outside world, so he can contemplate life. Furthermore, cigarettes also serve to 'de-charge' Hank: he smoked a lot more during the open exam when pressure was high, and that is also when he became really addicted to smoking; he had a few moments of smoking alone at the harbour when he broke up with his girlfriend; he immediately reaches out for a cigarette when he is wronged or gets angry.

A note on the researcher's subjective emotional experience after the interviews with Hank: despite the openness displayed by Hank, the researcher felt that Hank's demeanour was covered by a layer of darkness. This might be due to the traumatic experiences in early infancy, and how his life story developed afterwards; including expulsion from school and the betrayal of his girlfriend and best friend. The researcher had a nightmare after the first interview with Hank. She dreamt that something had caught fire in the basement of her apartment, and she had to run for her life. This made her wonder if that is how Hank has been feeling all this time, that, is, running away from something that is on fire in his unconscious.

Anthony: a young man with extremely long hair

Anthony is a 21-year-old final year student majoring in Business Administration at university. Anthony came into the interview room wearing an artist's hat and very fashionable clothing. He also wore his hair long, which is quite unusual for men in Hong Kong. Later on, he mentioned that the bachelor's degree he is studying has no honours, and he got into this programme indirectly via different interim schools, instead of straight from high school, and it is clear from our conversation that he is not confident of finding a decent job after graduation; he was also worried that his long hair might give a bad impression to potential employers.

Anthony is the younger of the two boys in his family. His brother is six years older and the two of them are very close, even though his brother no longer lives with him and their parents. His brother did not go to university and, according to Anthony, his brother looks and behaves very differently from Anthony. Anthony's father works nightshifts, so he rarely sees his sons, and his mother has been a full-time housewife since she married their father. Anthony said that he loves old stuff; he is a very nostalgic person and does not want anyone to 'touch' his childhood memories. For instance, he won a Disney piglet stuffed toy with a bell at the AIA Carnival when he was five or six years old, and even today he still keeps the toy at his bedside and cuddles it every night. The soft toy is worn with age, but he has only washed it once or twice in the past 15 years fearing that too much washing would cause damage to his piglet toy, and that it would lose its eyes, ears, mouth, and nose. He would also cry if that happened to his toy.

Anthony started smoking regularly at 17 years old when he was under a lot of pressure studying for his open examination. He picked up smoking under the influence of his girlfriend at that time. He regarded smoking as a very 'comfortable action', so comfortable that words fail to explain it. It is not a physical comfort, but more like a psychological comfort, something that gives him an excuse to rest and take breaks. He likes to smoke with his friends for social bonding, and when he smokes alone, he usually uses cigarettes to pass his time, especially when he is in between things, or waiting for a bus and has nothing to do, for example, when he starts to feel lonely. Smoking is seen as a habitual 'action' in order to keep himself company, and a cigarette is something that makes him feel less lonely, very similar to the role of a pet. He also loves to smoke after meals, because it gives him a very comfortable feeling, and he feels that a meal is not complete without the cigarette.

He also spoke of the recently and highly distressing breakup with his girlfriend. Apart from talking to friends, he mainly used cigarettes to cope with the separation. His most disappointing cigarette was the one that smelled and tasted completely different from his regular one. He suspected that the cigarette was dated, and he got rid of the entire pack immediately after smoking only half a stick, despite the high price of cigarettes in Hong Kong. His favourite cigarette was the one that he smoked after his open exam when he knew that he had done well enough to secure a place at university, and that he could therefor take a break from studying and exams for a little while.

Anthony smokes for time out, to relieve exhaustion and stress, and for companionship. Also, 'time out' is an important smoking moment for Anthony, as he mentioned more a few times that cigarettes give him an opportunity to take breaks, something that he always looks forward to. Whenever he feels exhausted or overwhelmed by work or his study, he will always reach for a smoke, which allows him to relax and not think about anything else for a short while. Finally, cigarettes help Anthony to 'de-charge' and are a stress relief function after finishing a project or after an exam, which make him feel comfortable and relaxed. Anthony also expressed that he usually has a very strong desire to smoke whenever he is unhappy, like breaking up with his girlfriends. A cigarette is like a loyal companion who is always there for him no matter how he feels.

Holly: a new immigrant from mainland China

Holly is a 20-year-old, Year 2 university student in Hong Kong. When asked to introduce herself, she mentioned spontaneously that she is an immigrant from mainland China and only came to Hong Kong when she was ten, which is a secret she has been keeping from her classmates and friends (note: mainland Chinese immigrants are usually discriminated against by the local Hong Kong people, they are often the target of bullying and social isolation at school, especially for immigrants who come from outside the Guangdong Province where Mandarin is spoken, not Cantonese, the language spoken by the Hong Kong people.) After a brief moment of silence, she continued and said that she is two years older than her classmates in the same class, because she repeated one year in Grade 5 and another year in Grade 11 due to her bad conduct and grades. Holly felt the gap between her and her Hong Kong classmates was not only because of her older age but also because, generally speaking, she does not like Hong Kong people. Holly thinks that they are very mean and cold compared to mainland Chinese people, and she does not want her Hong Kong friends to know that she is from mainland China. Because of that, Holly has always felt strange and out of place in Hong Kong, and yet she does not want to get in touch with her old mainland Chinese friends, because she also feels inferior to those locals who have their own houses.

Holly is the only child in her family and stayed with her mother in Dong Guan in China before moving to Hong Kong. Her father is a cross-border truck driver between Hong Kong and China, he works a night shift, so he is usually not at home one day per week. Her mother used to be a full-time housewife when they still lived in China, but she hardly looked after Holly due to her preoccupations with her own social life. After she moved to Hong Kong two years ago, Holly's mother started working as a dishwasher at the Hong Kong Jockey Club, and she used most of her salary to pay for Holly's tuition in Hong Kong.

Holly started smoking when she was 12 years old under the influence of a group of friends she met through an online gaming community. Holly felt excluded from her friends being the only non-smoker in the group, so she decided to buy her first cigarette in secret to find out how it felt like to smoke. From then onwards, Holly fell in love with smoking and she has been unable to separate herself from cigarettes, as her heart would convulse and beat faster if she could not smoke. She did not tell any Hong Kong classmates that she smoked due to social pressure, as smoking is seen as a bad habit.

A cigarette is like a toy or mobile phone to Holly, something that she wants to have around her all the time, something that she would feel extremely agitated about if it were absent. Her favourite cigarette was Marlboro Ice Blast (her regular brand) which she smoked immediately after crossing the Hong Kong border the day before our interview, when she went to China with her friend. Holly had been seriously deprived of smoking when she ran out of cigarettes at home the night before the trip. She could not find her regular Marlboro Ice Blast brand on the China side, so she was offered a Capri Superslims cigarette by her friend, which was a complete disappointment and made her feel 'unstable' and 'unsafe', as she described that cigarette as 'hopeless'. She felt 'awesome' after finally getting to smoke her regular brand after she went back to the Hong Kong border, which was a 'real cigarette' in her opinion. Her most disappointing cigarette was the one she smoked inside her friend's car, which made her feel very dizzy and stuffy, and she came to the conclusion that she would feel extremely uncomfortable smoking in a dark and suffocating entrapped environment. Holly has an inseparable relationship with her cigarettes; her strong desire to smoke when her cigarettes are not available is like her heart being clutched, which only makes her desire stronger. There was a time when she was rushing and knew that she was already late for school, and she suddenly had an urge to smoke a cigarette as a consolation, after knowing she would be late for school anyway, but she had run out, so she approached a stranger to ask for a cigarette. She compared her desire to smoke to her longing to see a boyfriend whom she had not seen for a long time.

Cigarettes are very multi-purposed for Holly, as she uses cigarettes in the 'time out' moments when she decides to enjoy her smoke off campus, as a consolation, in order to take her away from the stressful awareness that she was late for school. She also uses cigarettes to 'de-charge', when she manages to achieve a sense of calmness and stability by smoking her regular cigarette brand after the poor experience of smoking an extremely disappointing cigarette, an experience that made her feel unstable and unsafe. Holly always has cigarettes around her, as she believes that smoking enables her to feel more settled, restored, and recharged, so the 're-vive' function of smoking also exists for Holly.

A note on the researcher's subjective emotional experience after the interviews with Holly: the researcher had a dream about her oldest school friend with whom she had a profound disagreement. The distress and long-term effect made her feel as if her entire high school days were obliterated because of it. This may well mirror the helplessness experienced by Holly when she had to part with her more genuine friends in mainland China as she moved to Hong Kong with her family.

Anita: a child who grew up in a foster family due to the poverty of her biological parents

Anita is a 21-year-old final year student majoring in Business Administration. Anita was born in Indonesia and moved to Hong Kong when she was five. Anita is the only child of Indonesian Chinese parents. Her parents were both very poor, and they had to go to work every day, leaving no time to look after Anita. Because of that, Anita was 'given away' to her wealthy aunt (her father's younger sister) and uncle as a god-daughter when she was a baby, so she literally grew up in her uncle and aunt's big house and rarely saw her biological parents throughout her childhood. During these the years, Anita developed a strong and deep relationship with her adoptive parents. She still remembers how she looked at her Indonesian adoptive father every day in his office through the side stream as he exhaled smoke from his cigarette, the aromatic tobacco smell emanating from him, and how her adoptive mother bathed her every day until she was quite grown up, and the warmth and sense of security she felt when she was held in her adoptive parents' arms. According to Anita, when she was five years old, she was suddenly taken away ('kidnapped') by her biological parents from her Indonesian adoptive parents, and afterwards the whole family moved to Hong Kong. Anita's father worked in a bank as an errand boy in Hong Kong, but lost his job when Anita was nine years old. In her father's words, he was 'replaced by computers' and has been unemployed ever since. Anita's mother is a masseuse and a beautician, she used to have a shop in a commercial building, now runs a private (illegal) facial parlour at home.

In Anita's recollection, she was not happy at school and did not have many friends. Most of her classmates were from wealthy families, so she felt very distant from them. She also attributed her lack of good friends to her parents' unwillingness to socialise with her classmates' families, especially in her primary school days.

Anita started smoking when she was 15 years old. At that time, she met a group of friends at school who taught her how to smoke and drink. She started skipping school and not returning home. She admitted that her behaviour had caused her parents a great deal of distress at that time. Cigarettes have the power to bring back fond memories of her childhood in Indonesia, when she was still the adored daughter of her Indonesian adoptive parents. Her Indonesian father smoked a kretek (clove) cigarette brand called Dji Sam Soe 234, which has a unique and aromatic smell. Even now, Anita still loves to light the same Dji Sam Soe 234 cigarette and let it burn, whenever she can get hold of one. She loves to smell the smoke of the cigarette to remind her of the happy times she spent with her adoptive father, and the security she felt. This particular brand of cigarette produces smoke that soothes Anita whenever she is unhappy. Although she was promised a shop from her rich adoptive Indonesian parents, they turned their back on Anita after the birth of their biological grandchildren a few years ago. Anita felt extremely hurt and disappointed, and she still does not understand how people can change so drastically and suddenly, and why her adoptive parents would so readily turn their back on her. Anita considers cigarettes to have an equal value with friends, as they both give her a sense of security. However, the only difference being that, unlike friends who can abandon Anita at any moment they wish, cigarettes will not leave her, only she has the power to leave them. To Anita, a cigarette is a very good icebreaker with strangers, and it also serves the dual function of providing relaxation and restoration. The smoke produced by a cigarette is a carrier for bad stuff, and smoking is a distillation process to filter out the bad stuff through exhalation, leaving only the good stuff inside the body. Despite her fondness for smoking, she also regards the inhaled smoke as dangerous, and she stated explicitly that she does not want the inhaled smoke to have direct contact with her stomach, which is also why she would never smoke with an empty stomach, the latter reason being more psychological than physiological in meaning for her.

The single most important smoking moment for Anita is the highly personal 'de-charge' moment for stress relief and achievement of inner balance: smoking during breaks is an enjoyment, as it helps her exhale fatigue and grudges from customers. Smoking also gives her time to think things over and through, especially when she is stressed. The recent ideal cigarette, which she mentioned in the interview, was the one she smoked on campus, a smoke that made her feel very relaxed after a stressful day at school. She loves to sniff the Dji Sam Soe 234 kretek cigarette for soothing purposes when she is unhappy, and she enjoys watching the burning ciga-rette producing a still and calm line of white smoke, which reminds her of the good old days when she watched her Indonesian adoptive father smoking it in his office at home. Anita always smokes when she is unhappy; she sees the cigarette smoke as a way to remove all the bad stuff, leaving only the good stuff inside her, as all the bad stuff is extracted in the exhalation process. Closely linked to the 'de-charge' moment is the 'revive' smoking moment that Anita spoke of in the interviews, where the tobacco smell that stays in her hand after finishing each cigarette made her feel secured and restored. She also actively uses cigarettes in the 'time out' mo-ment when she wants to have a short period of isolation from the world, like sitting on a massage chair relaxing completely, as she put it.

Cooper: the youngest sibling who needs to shoulder the entire family's financial burden

Cooper is a 20-year-old, Year 1 student majoring in Hotel Management. Cooper grew up in a single-parent family. Her parents quarrelled all the time in her child-hood and her father ran away after a row with her mother when she was in pri-mary school, leaving her mother, her elder sister, and her living alone together. Cooper still remembers that the row was about her school textbook fee, so she has always felt extremely guilty about her parents' quarrel, believing she was the one who caused their separation. Her father went to Italy after the separation but was returned to Hong Kong by immigration authorities; he later disappeared again. Her father never actively got in touch with the three of them, and sometimes he would just suddenly show up for a while and then disappear again. Cooper does not know where her father is, nor does she miss him, because she is very used to living with her mother and sister, just the three of them, without needing a father. In fact, she even mentioned explicitly that she prefers her father not to come back to their life anymore. The only thing she remembers of her father was that he fre-quently beat her and her sister for small things in the past; there was a time when she was six or seven years old when she tried to fight back but ended up being lifted up by the arm and beaten even harder and then thrown off by her father. He only stopped when her mother came and rescued her. In Cooper's memory, her mother only beat her once, when she found out that she smoked. Other than that, one of the happiest moments in her life was when her mother took her and her sister to Disneyland when she was 12, and the three had a lot of fun together. Cooper also enjoys spending time with her mother alone, without her sister. She recalled a time when she was the only one helping her mother deliver the goods to the shop, a task that her sister was too lazy to do, and Cooper enjoyed the vanity of being seen as the only useful, helpful and adored daughter of her mother. Cooper's mother works in the Chinese medicine wholesaling business, but her income fluctuates. Cooper's elder sister is unemployed and relies on her boyfriend to support her financially. She behaves like a little princess at home and is highly addicted to costume play and TV games, she has been emotionally unstable since her father ran away and has a disposition to violence. For example, three years ago, when their mother refused to give her sister money since she herself also had no money, her sister lost her temper and started to smash and hit things at home, and she also physically attacked her mother, injuring her mouth. When she was little, and the family still had a maid, her sister lost control and threatened the maid with a knife. Cooper could influence her sister's behaviour during the argument and her mother did not want to make a big fuss about it, so they let go of the incident. Cooper works part-time in the finance industry while she is studying, so she is the only one supporting her family financially and she always feels pressured by this heavy burden on her shoulders. She does not like to stay home and prefers to hang out with friends, because her mother and sister always ask her for money whenever she is at home.

Cooper had a very unsteady and fragmented high school life. She was transferred from one school to another seven times during her high school years: after repeating Form 2 for three years, Cooper was finally expelled from her first high school when she was 15 years old. After that, she left school and ran away from home to stay with her best friend who had also been expelled from school. During that year away from home, she simply hung out and played with her friend every day, and she moved back home only after her friend lost a place to stay. After three years of idleness, one day she suddenly realised that she did not want to follow her mother and elder sister's footsteps. Because of her interrupted and sporadic high school life when she was a teenager, Cooper was not able to establish any stable and meaningful friendships with any of her classmates, and she feels that there is always a generation gap with them due to her older age and the working experience that her classmates lack.

Cooper spoke of the first smoke in the morning as the most satisfying cigarette of the whole day, a cigarette that she needs desperately to wake her up. To Cooper, smoking is like 'blowing out' all the bad emotions, it makes her feel that she is not alone; a cigarette is like 'food for her mind', it is an object that will never disappoint or abandon her, both in happy and difficult times. She never finishes smoking the entire cigarette when she is happy; she enjoys lighting one cigarette after the other, and she only smokes half of each cigarette and stubs it out and lights another. This action of lighting and stubbing out one cigarette after the other makes her feel

strangely satisfied. On the contrary, she will definitely smoke out the entire cigarette when she is not happy, a behaviour that she is aware of but never understands.
Cooper regards the cigarette's role as similar to that of her mother, someone who is
always there with her when she needs her but easily forgotten when she has other
distractions or friends around. Related to the mothering role of the cigarette, she
also finds the cigarette smoke to be highly protective against the external environment, as she used the cigarette smoke as a protective shield against her boyfriend
when they quarrelled: she chain-smoked and kept blowing out the smoke, so he
could not get near her. Cooper is very sensitive to critical looks when she smokes;
her fear of judging eyes or attracting any kind of attention is so overwhelming that
she does not even dare to call out to hail a bus. She feels that her voice is strange
and somewhat hoarse, and she admitted that she lacks the confidence to listen to her
own recorded voice, although it remains unknown whether this belief has anything
to do with her parents' incessant quarrelling in her childhood. Overall, she has no
confidence that drivers will stop the bus at her request, so she always waits for
others to do it, sometimes ending up walking for hours back home if nobody calls
out to stop it! Cooper always has a nauseous feeling when she smokes, but instead
of hating it, she loves the sensation of taking out something from her mouth. That
is also one of the reasons why she loves to smoke cigarettes, in order for her to
have that nauseous sensation. At the end of the second interview, she revealed to
the researcher that she always gets oesophageal bleeding resulting from frequent
self-induced vomiting.

Cooper smokes mainly to 'de-charge', especially in emotionally difficult moments: she has a habit of chain-smoking whenever she is unhappy, for example,
when breaking up with her boyfriend. Smoking cigarettes makes her feel that she
is capable of blowing out all the bad emotions, so she does not have to think about
them anymore, and she is no longer alone because her cigarette is her constant
companion, a companion who will always be there for her. She also chain-smokes
when she is happy. She feels like doing something with her hand, so she just lights
one cigarette after another without smoking the entire cigarette. Cooper went for
a smoke immediately after a chaotic presentation, and that cigarette was regarded
by her as her favourite cigarette of the day, as she felt extremely relieved after
the smoke, as if nothing concerned her anymore and she could finally have a moment to calm down and restore her inner balance. Another important moment for
smoking is the 'time out' moment, where Cooper intentionally uses the blown-out
smoke from her cigarette to form a smoke screen, in order to shield herself from a
boyfriend during a fight.

A note on the researcher's subjective emotional experience after the interviews
with Cooper: compared to other respondents, it took much longer for Cooper to
warm up to the interviewer. She was reserved and spoke very little at the beginning.
As rapport developed during the interview, there was a dramatic change in behaviour and she did not seem to want to leave. Even after the researcher indicated
repeatedly that the interview was over, Cooper stayed on for another 25 minutes.

After the first interview, the researcher felt unusually hungry and she ate a lot at dinner afterwards. This was very out of character for the researcher as she normally skips dinner. She wonders if it has anything to do with Cooper's revelation that she experiences oesophageal bleeding due to frequent self-induced vomiting. Perhaps this reflects an unconscious wish for Cooper to stop vomiting and start taking in more nourishment.

Emerald: a girl who was sexually molested by her divorced mother's live-in boyfriend

Emerald is a 23-year-old recent university graduate majoring in Commercial Translation. She used to live in Kuala Lumpur and only came to Hong Kong for university studies four years ago when she was 19 years old.

Emerald's parents were separated when she was three years old, and her mother obtained custody of Emerald and her elder sister who is two years older. Despite fighting hard for custody, her mother was very career minded and she preferred to hang out with friends rather than looking after her daughters at home. For convenience and personal comfort, she sent Emerald and her sister to Kuala Lumpur to live with their grandmothers, and in Emerald's words, her mother 'dumped' them. Emerald felt that her mother did not really care much about her and her sister, as evident in the careless and sloppy way she took care of them. On the contrary, Emerald felt that they were treated very well by their grandmothers and all their relatives in Kuala Lumpur. Her mother rarely visited them in Kuala Lumpur; at most she would just make long distance calls to chat with the sisters for a while whenever she felt like it. In order to make up for lost bonding time, from the age of seven or eight years old, Emerald and her sister would usually return to Hong Kong for a month at the end of every year to visit their mother. There is a lack of emotional attachment between Emerald and her mother, as Emerald believes that her mother was very irresponsible for leaving her and her sister in Kuala Lumpur. When she was 13 years old, she even told her mother straight to her face, in a very calm manner, that it would be impossible for her to compensate for the horrible things she had done to her daughters years ago, and that she has no feelings for her mother, even though she would still provide for her mother in old age; but she cannot love her because her mother does not deserve it. Her mother used to live with a boyfriend in Hong Kong, and Emerald revealed to the researcher that when she came to live with her mother during the summer holidays, she was sexually abused by this man when she was only 15 years old. After a few years, when Emerald moved back to Hong Kong permanently, she kicked this man out of their home by changing the door locks while her mother was out of town, and she helped her mother to divorce him. Emerald has never been close to her father, nor her father's family in Hong Kong.

Emerald smoked her first cigarette when she was 16 years old under the influence of a friend she met through Facebook, but she stopped smoking after that first stick because she felt the disapproval of a mother and her baby on the street when she smoked. When she was 18, she broke up with her boyfriend, and she started to work part-time in a bar where everybody smoked, so she picked it up again. To Emerald, cigarettes take her to a world where she can rest and enjoy a brief moment of quietness and peace. A cigarette is most important to her when she is unhappy. It calms her down when she is angry, and it stops her from venting her anger at other people, therefore a cigarette is a medium for stress absorption and it has a cushioning and stress relief function for her. At the end of the second interview, Emerald revealed to the researcher that the friend who gave her the first cigarette was actually a tomboy in love with her at that time, and she associates smoking with romantic love instead of friendship, because a cigarette is seen as a substitute for a lover who is willing to spend time with her and console her sadness at times. A cigarette is also compliant and available, allowing Emerald to use it any time, like her own mother who let her do whatever she wanted. She smokes less these days since she started practising yoga a year and a half ago, and in fact, at the time of the interview, she was about to obtain her yoga instructor's licence.

Emerald spoke of her most satisfying cigarette as the one she smoked a day before the interview, when she knew she had passed her motor vehicle written exam, and after she had seen her aunt off at the airport (she was not able to smoke freely during her aunt's visit, not wanting her aunt to know that she smoked). The smoke was extremely comfortable and relaxing, almost like the sensation of stretching after a yoga practice. This is what smoking can do to Emerald: transport her to a world with short moments of quietness and peace, a world where she can finally take a rest. Emerald had the most disappointing cigarette just before the interview. As she stood beside a rubbish bin on the street to have a quick smoke before she came up to the interview room, she felt that she was being stared at by people on the street, and she was also preoccupied with being caught by the police when she threw the cigarette butt on the ground, so she quickly dragged a few puffs, discarded the cigarette and quickly left.

The two most important smoking moments for Emerald are the 'time out' and 'de-charge' moments. Her 'time out' moments include sitting alone in an outdoor café, smoking a cigarette while observing passers-by. She uses this brief smoking moment to detach herself from reality and assume the role of a bystander, so she can steal a short moment of rest in a peaceful place. She also likes to stand still when she smokes on the street in order to better isolate herself, so that she can observe people and things more clearly. On a trip to Thailand with friends, she stole a private moment to smoke alone after swimming, away from a noisy non-smoking travel companion, where she enjoyed the space, the peace and the quietness, and she was grateful that there was nobody there to disturb her, finally. To Emerald, a cigarette is a soother and a buffer that has a cushioning and stress relief function when she is very unhappy and angry. It helps her absorb her tantrums and stops her from taking it out on others, and she uses cigarettes to transform her anger and sorrow into calmness when she has just had a fight with her boyfriend or she has been rejected by someone who she likes.

Abyss: a handsome young man who was born prematurely and began life in an incubator

Abyss is a 21-year-old, Year 1 student majoring in Image Design in a college in Hong Kong. When Abyss was born, the doctor suspected that he had Down's syndrome because he displayed some of the symptoms. He also had a low birth weight, and was put into the incubator for a period of time before being released from hospital. Abyss was told by his grandmother that at that time, his mother's sister came to the hospital and told the whole world that baby Abyss was an oaf because his palm lines were broken off! Abyss still hates his aunt for this remark born of superstition.

Abyss's parents separated when he was three and were divorced when he was six. Since then, Abyss had been living with his grandmother and father in Hong Kong. He has a very poor relationship with his mother, actually detesting her, so he has never spent time with her and only saw her occasionally when she 'dropped by for free meals.' Abyss also remembered very well that when he was two to three years old, his mother slapped him hard on the face for using bad language on a school bus. While unwilling to do so, a few years ago, in order to resume his studies at university, he began to live with his mother in Hong Kong. His father had already re-married and moved to China. Despite being beaten brutally as a child every time his father returned home drunk in the middle of the night, or when he was kicked out of kindergarten when he was six years old and also out of high school, Abyss still admires his father, saying that he is the most talented designer in the world, and he proudly told the researcher that his father is the design director of a well-known company in China.

Abyss was expelled from school for the second time when he was in Grade 10 at the age of 15, after being caught smoking on campus a few times and taking almost half his class to an illegal rave party he organised. After he was expelled from school, he worked as a full-time party organiser, with an income based on the total number of invited people who attend parties. He managed to earn a lot of money at that time, sometimes up to more than HK$100,000 per month, as a result of his connections. However, he decided to leave the industry after two years as law enforcement by the police started to tighten, leaving no room for him to organise large-scale parties which often contravened safety regulations. He was then sent to a boarding school in China by his father. However, he did not like China and he felt very stressed studying there due to the cultural differences between him and his classmates. Abyss ended up burning himself out after two years, so he was sent back to Hong Kong to continue with his tertiary education.

Abyss had his first cigarette when he was 15 years old under the influence of a group of Western boys and American-Chinese classmates with whom he socialised at an international school. He also coughed badly and did not enjoy the experience. However, he accepted the cigarette the second time he was offered it in order not to feel excluded as he wanted desperately to fit in. All of his friends smoked and there little else he could do while they were smoking. From then onwards, he became 'severely addicted' to smoking, as he put it himself, and he grinds his teeth if there is no cigarette, or when he has no money to buy cigarettes. He has a strong desire to smoke, a desire that is similar to an insatiable hunger and can never be satisfied no matter how much he smokes.

Abyss thinks the first cigarette in the morning is always the most satisfying smoke, and he is obsessed with having a cigarette first thing in the morning on an empty stomach. To him, cigarettes are like his mental food, and he will go a long way to ensure that he has his morning smoke. He likes to chain smoke and thinks that smoking magnifies his emotions and feelings, both happy and sad.

There are two smoking moments when Abyss indulges in chain-smoking: the 'time out' and the 'de-charge' moments. Abyss will chain smoke when he wants to get into thinking mode, and the cigarette helps him enter this 'thinking world', while observing outside reality at the same time. When his brain is at war and replete with many chaotic ideas, smoking helps him to isolate himself from this insecure world instantly, very much like finding a hole to retreat into, or hiding beneath a blanket to isolate himself from the outside world. In the 'de-charge' moment, cigarettes play a significant role when he is anxious and unhappy: he chain-smokes when he is not happy, and holding a cigarette makes him feel more secure and calm. Cigarettes also help contain his anxieties and soothe him when he feels apprehensive, for example, when he was trying to borrow money from his friends to pay off his credit card bill.

A note on the researcher's subjective emotional experience after interviews with Abyss: despite a problematic and disruptive childhood, Abyss is a mature and charming person. He would be highly employable as a brand ambassador. He talked in a confident and charismatic way. The researcher wondered how a boy with such a traumatic childhood could become the person he is today. Is the real Abyss hidden behind a mask? The researcher had a dream after the first interview: a zombie was with the researcher's mother on the other side of a door. The researcher was desperate to feed her mother, so she negotiated with the zombie and asked him to feed her mother on her behalf. The zombie agreed but the researcher was still very scared of the zombie. Does the zombie represent a part of Abyss? Is Abyss conflicted between feeding and killing her mother?

Samuel: an athlete, nursed and raised by his grandmother

Samuel is a 21-year-old, final year student majoring in Business Studies in a Hong Kong university. Samuel was nursed by his grandmother, because both his parents had to work and had no time to look after him. Samuel was always sent to China during the summer holidays with his grandmother, so he was taught by his mother to take long-haul buses alone, and how to take care of his illiterate grandmother at just six years old. His mother started her own business as the owner of a cleaning company when Samuel was in Grade 5, aged 11, and she started to come home later and later every night because of work. Samuel's parents were divorced in the same year, and he had some memories of his parents quarrelling and his mother crying frequently, but those memories are quite blurry as he was very young when that happened. After the divorce, Samuel chose to stay with his mother and moved to a new apartment, as his mother had managed to save enough to buy her own apartment. At that time, he did not understand what divorce meant, and he simply thought that his parents lived in different places and it was no big deal to him. In fact, he even felt happy as he could play TV games at his mother's apartment, and football at his father's home. When he entered Grade 7, Samuel began to notice the difference between him and his classmates and wondered why his classmates lived with both their parents at home. He sought counselling from his class teacher, and he finally understood what divorce actually meant: that when two people stop loving each other, they would be better off separating from each other.

Samuel was a very active boy and he played a lot of sports including basketball, football, and volleyball on the school teams in high school. Samuel injured his knees in Grade 9, the same year he had to sit for the open examination. Knowing that being a professional athlete in Hong Kong was not a viable career option, he let go of his dream, took advice from his family, and gave up all sports after the knee injury. He now only plays football occasionally.

Samuel started smoking in Grade 8, accepting a cigarette after being offered one three times. At first, he only smoked after his training sessions, perhaps a few sticks a month, as he was afraid that his mother would find out about him smoking. He started to smoke more frequently when he began working part-time in Grade 10. For Samuel, smoking makes him feel soothed and satisfied, and sleepy at times, similar to the sensation after a large and satisfying meal. Cigarettes give him a momentary feeling of extreme satisfaction without all the discomforts. This smoking moment belongs to Samuel completely; time suddenly stops, the world disappears when he smokes, and the cigarette becomes an ideal companion making this quiet and ideal world perfect for him, so in a way, for Samuel, smoking is very much like sleeping. Samuel also associates smoking a cigarette with finishing a task and accomplishing something. A cigarette is similar to a person who is willing to help him, he does not like to waste a cigarette, and he would rather miss the bus and wait for another than stub out a half-finished cigarette.

Samuel likes the softness of the cigarette, and he always smokes after a full meal, and he smokes very slowly to savour the lingering sensation. Samuel spoke of his most enjoyable smoke as the one when he was on holiday in Japan with his friends, when they loitered on the balcony watching the sunset facing the ocean, as smoking while watching the open sea always gives him a heightened sense of relaxation and enjoyment.

The two most prominent smoking moments for Samuel are the 'time out' and 'de-charge' moments. In the 'time out' moments, Samuel loves to smoke alone at home quietly, doing nothing, and thinking of nothing. Time seems to stop, and that moment belongs to him completely, and a cigarette makes the world complete to him in that special space. Sitting by the seaside and watching the sunset alone was a very surreal and yet enjoyable experience, and he felt very content in those few minutes and the world looked perfect to him. In Samuel's 'de-charge' moments, a cigarette soothes him when he is under pressure, so he always uses cigarettes to de-stress. He usually smokes for relaxation purposes after a journey, or when he has finished writing an important paper for school. When he gets agitated and annoyed, he uses cigarettes to calm him down, and he always smokes during school recess to feel recharged and restored.

A note on the researcher's subjective emotional experience after the interviews with Samuel: the researcher felt unusually tired during the entire interview with Samuel. Her eyelids were so heavy that they almost closed. For a few moments, the researcher felt that her mind was wandering, almost falling asleep in the interview. This made the researcher wonder if it was Samuel's way of telling her how sleepy and relaxed he felt when he smoked his cigarettes.

Chapter 15

Spotting the 'regressive' smoking moments

Commercial research conducted by the tobacco industry is based on a conscious level of processing, therefore it is of limited use to our present discussion. However, it is worth noting that out of the eight smoking moments, only two are related to the social moments of smoking, the remaining six are all related to the personal moments of smoking, and amongst these six personal moments, there are two where tobacco use is the 'core agent' driving smokers' behaviour, where they have a high engagement level with their cigarettes: these are the 'me-time' and the 'relax' moments. It is also interesting to observe that these two moments account for the lion's share of 30 to 50 per cent respectively of all smoking moments globally, indicating the importance and prevalence of these two highly personal moments of cigarette consumption. Both personal moments involve a temporary detachment from external reality and a fluid movement between internal and external reality, two important characteristics that have been completely ignored by commercial research within the tobacco industry, whose focus is more on the extraction of insight based on a conscious level of functioning. These distinctive and unique 'regressive' characteristics of the 'me-time' and 'relax' moments reveal a whole new world of meanings from a psychoanalytic perspective.

There are many triggers and moments for smoking, but not all are regressive ones in which smokers display an increased level of regressive behaviour or feel these to be very special moments. Our objective was to identify smoking moments that were 'regressive' in nature, moments that move away from mature to more primitive levels of functioning, moments that are characterised by the infantile merged state and the concreteness of the smokers' thinking and behaviours, and moments that move away from the reality principle towards the pleasure principle. The above three criteria help us to separate the 'regressive' smoking moments that are highly personal, from the 'non-regressive' smoking moments which are mainly concerned with the social aspect of smoking and other low involvement forms of the personal aspect of smoking. We do not claim that the cigarette is a regressed form of transitional object in moments of social

DOI: 10.4324/9781003329077-21

aspects which are 'non-regressive' in nature. In fact, what is interesting is how a cigarette becomes a regressed form of an infantile transitional object in the 'regressive' smoking moments that are highly personal in nature. Since this book is about Winnicott's transitional object aspect of cigarettes, our focus is on these very personal and 'regressive' moments of cigarette consumption that are characterised by:

1. **Regression to dependence,** to moments of infantile merging with the mother, and to moments of merging between the infant's lips and the mother's nipples, so that the smoker can re-experience the illusion of omnipotence. This is physically reinforced by the perceived merging between the smokers' lips and the filter of the cigarette when he smokes the cigarette. This sense of magical merging is further strengthened by the convenience of smoking, as the cigarettes are almost always located upon the smoker's person. This is also the moment where smokers move from a reality principle to a pleasure principle.
2. A highly **concrete relationship** between the smoker and his cigarettes, resembling an early stage of infantile relationship. This is the moment when the smoker interacts with the cigarettes in a very physical and bodily manner, which is different from an ordinary relationship with other people where facial expressions and words are used, rather than more tactile ones.
3. A **fluid sort of regression**, which means that the regressive moments kick in immediately whenever the smokers experience stressful feelings, so cigarette consumption is closely connected with the emotional state of the smoker. What is important here is the speed and the magical appearance of the cigarette whenever it is needed, which is strengthened by the physical convenience of carrying a pack of cigarettes in the smoker's pocket at all times; this is very similar to the magical appearance of the transitional object in the infant's world.

As summarised in Table 15.1, a total of eight smoking moments were identified by the commercial research undertaken by the tobacco industry, each of these moments is rooted in one core human need. These eight moments can be further divided into six personal smoking moments including 'pass the time' and 'me time' moments which are rooted in the core need of 'connection with self', 'self-reward' and 'relax' moments which are rooted in the core need of 'self-balance', 'focus/ problem solver' and 'boost/start up' moments which are rooted in the core need of 'performance'; the two social moments include 'projection of self' and 'socialise' moments which are both rooted in the core need of 'connection with others' (see also Part I, Chapter 2).

A comparison of the themes of the respondents' smoking moments with the tobacco industry's 'smoking moments' research suggests that out of the six highly

Table 15.1 Summary of respondents' smoking moments

	PERSONAL MOMENTS										SOCIAL MOMENTS		
	CONNECT WITH SELF			SELF BALANCE			PERFOMANCE				CONNECTING WITH OTHERS		
Moments	1a	1b		2a	2b		3a		3b		4a		4b
	Pass the time	Me Time		Self-reward	Relax		Focus/problem solver		Boost/start up		Projection of self		Socialise
Core needs	Occupy empty momentes	Time on my own		Indulge myself	Rebalancing myself		Concentraing and thoght process		Manage perfomance and energy levels		Control what others see of me		Bond and share
Types	**Pass the time**	**Time to be myself**	**Time out**	**Self-reward**	**De-charge**	**Revive**	**Focus**	**Problem solver**	**Boost**	**Satrt up**	**Impress**	**Blend in**	**Socialise**
Hark	1		2	1	4						1	1	4
Anthony	1		2	1	2							1	2
Holly	1		1	1	1	1			1			3	1
Anita	1		1		5	2	1		1			1	1
Cooper	1		1	2	3					1		1	1
Emerald			5		3	1	1		1			1	2
Abyss	1		2	1	2	1	1			1	1	1	1
Samuel			2	2	4		1		1			3	1

Note The numbers in the matrix indicate the number of occurrences of these smoking moments in the interviews.

personal smoking moments, two moments emerged consistently across all the eight respondents (see Table 15.1), which are as follows:

1. The '**time out**' sub-type under the '**me time**' moment where the respondents have a short period of isolation from the outside world, a short moment where they can be out of reach from overstimulation and free to be themselves.
2. The '**de-charge**' sub-type under the '**relax**' moment, where the respondents can enjoy a short duration of stress relief and inner balance restoration, a moment where they can calm themselves down from over-stimulation and feel soothed and back in control again.

All of the eight smoking moments (described in Chapter 2) contain signs of infantile merging with the mother and a concrete relationship between the smoker and his cigarettes, both of which are mainly driven by how cigarettes are physically consumed, that is, a merging of the smoker's lips and the filter of the cigarette, and a merging of the smoke with the smokers' body through inhalation and exhalation of the smoke, and a type of interaction that is highly tactile, physical, and bodily. However, only the 'time out' and 'de-charge' moments involve a fluid sort of regression and movements between internal and external realities triggered by stressful feelings of the smokers. This is an interesting piece of revelation that may not be of any interest to the tobacco industry, but it could contain important information and insight on the understanding of smoking addiction from a psychoanalytic perspective, especially when it comes to understanding the special qualities of these two personal moments of smoking and why they are different from the rest of the other six major smoking moments.

Smoking is an irrational behaviour, but smokers still continue to smoke despite consciously knowing the dangerous nature of cigarettes. From the above observations and analysis, we know that smoking is not just about peer influence or social pressure, but something very personal about the relationship between the smoker and the cigarette that goes beyond social pressure. Smoking is an intense and intimate experience between the smoker and their cigarettes. The fact that smokers continue to smoke despite knowing that cigarettes will kill them suggests that there must be unconscious forces behind the addiction, and this is where our research interest lies: to understand the unconscious forces behind smoking addiction. In the following chapter, we will move on to look at how Winnicott's model of the 'transitional object' and 'transitional phenomena' can help account for the unconscious motivations to perpetuate smoking addiction.

Chapter 16

The resemblance of a cigarette to the transitional object

A typical transitional object is a soft object within easy reach of the infant, usually part of a blanket, sheet, or other soft fabric used by the mother. The transitional object serves oral eroticism. This can be clearly seen in Cooper's interview when she said that the cigarette is an object that will never disappoint or abandon her, both in happy and sad moments, a cigarette is like food and nourishes her mind.

> … [a cigarette] keeps me company when I am alone. It helps me when I am unhappy, happy, or when I've had a full meal. It's around all these times, it helps me whenever I need it … happy and unhappy, I will smoke, I will keep smoking. Its role is to stand by me whenever I have quarrels with my folks, break up with my boyfriend, or go out drinking with my colleagues, all these occasions it is always next to me … it is food to my mind … it is feeding the needs of my mind.
>
> (Cooper, second interview)

In a certain way, the transitional object represents the mother. This was vividly demonstrated by Emerald when she equated a cigarette with a friend who let her use it, very much like her own mother, a mother whom she is very afraid of being too dependent on:

> … a cigarette is like a friend who always sits beside me, it won't talk to me, but it lets me use it and helps me relax. I also feel that it's quite mighty, it won't talk back, and it won't criticise me, but it would let me … I mean it devotes its whole life to me, lets me burn it all to ashes, in that sense it is really quite mighty …
>
> … I was scared of it when I used to smoke too much … it's the fear that I would become … I mean more and more dependent on it in the long run! Because when I light my cigarette by myself, it would sit beside me, I feel comfortable when it sits beside me when I am unhappy, but I don't want to be dependent on it! I don't want to be always detached from the reality and indulge in smoking everyday … I have to control myself, like using external measures such as not buying it, or not putting it in my pocket. And you can't ask for too many puffs from your friends' cigarettes, I will feel embarrassed. That's why I have to use this kind of external measures to reduce the dependence.
>
> (Emerald, second interview)

DOI: 10.4324/9781003320077-22

The transitional object is something that is 'created' by the baby between four to twelve months of age. It must be perceived by the baby as its own creation and cannot be prescribed by the mother directly, even though in reality it is given by the mother indirectly. When the baby is able to walk, it insists on taking it everywhere. The object retains the smell of the baby and the mother and it must not be washed; the baby would experience extreme distress if the object were to be misplaced, taken away, or lost. The baby becomes attached to the transitional object, and it is demanded when the baby is about to go to sleep or at times of stress, when the object will be pressed against the baby's face and mouth or is sucked. From waking to sleeping, the infant jumps from an objectively perceived world to a subjectively apperceived and self-created world. In between these two worlds there is a neutral territory in which all kinds of transitional phenomena take place. The infant uses the transitional object to bridge these two states, which explains why there is a strong need of the transitional object, particularly at the time of going to sleep, when the infant is dwelling in this intermediate area. This can be seen in Samuel's remarks in the second interview on how a cigarette made him feel. Samuel compared cigarettes with alcohol and said that cigarettes made him feel soft and peaceful, unlike alcohol which is heroic and masculine, the cigarette is the quiet type:

> … it (a cigarette) is kind of soft, a cigarette makes me feel soft, gives me a sense of peacefulness, it belongs to the quiet type … liquor, on the contrary, is very masculine and heroic. The ambiance I like is the quiet type, so I need something soft to go with me, then I will feel satisfied …
>
> (Samuel, second interview)

> … when you get to a place which is quiet, like the seaside, or the peak, the country park, you feel so relaxed, so comfy, the whole body is unwounded, then you will get that 'the world has stopped' feeling when you smoke.
>
> (Samuel, second interview)

When asked about what else would make him feel as relaxed as smoking a cigarette, Samuel immediately replied that it was sleeping!

Winnicott (1953) outlined seven special qualities in the relationship between the infant and the transitional object, which includes the infant assuming rights over the object; the object being affectionately loved as well as excitedly hated; the absolute unchangeable nature of the object unless it is changed by the infant; the survival of the object after instinctual loving and destruction; the object being perceived by the infant as having a life of its own; the location of the object being in an intermediate space between the internal and external reality; and its fate to lose meaning and its importance over time as the infant grows up.

1. The infant assumes rights over the object …
2. The object is affectionately cuddled as well as excitedly loved and mutilated.
3. It must never be changed, unless changed by the infant.

4. It must survive instinctual loving, and also hating …
5. Yet it must seem to the infant to give warmth, or to move, or to have texture, or to do something that seems to show it has vitality or reality of its own.
6. It comes from without from our point of view, but not so from the point of view of the baby. Neither does it come from within …
7. Its fate is to be gradually allowed to be decathected, so that in the course of years it becomes not so much forgotten as relegated to limbo …

(Winnicott, 1953, p. 91)

A closer look at the similarities between a cigarette and transitional object

Amongst the seven qualities listed out by Winnicott, the two most definitive qualities that differentiate a transitional object from a regular soothing object are the illusion of its vitality and liveliness, something that seems to have a life and reality of its own, and the location of the transitional object, which is neither from within nor from without, but in the intermediate area. The significance of these two qualities is also reflected in the interview results, as is seen in the fifth and sixth quality described by Winnicott, appearing consistently in all the interviews of the eight respondents (see Table 16.1).

The two-stage interview design is created to build rapport and establish a preliminary read in the first interview, followed by a second interview to build on the specifics mentioned in the first interview. Some respondents maintained a very conservative stance by speaking as superficially and as little as possible in the first interview, and were only willing to reveal more in the second interview after a prolonged warm-up and efforts to build rapport and trust by the researcher; some revealed a significant amount of private information to the researcher even in the first interviews. Hence, a different level of detail and information was obtained in each of these interviews across different respondents, rendering it unnecessary to split the results based on a different stage of the interviews. This approach was adopted by Hollway and Jefferson (2013).

Table 16.1 The presence of the specific quality of the transitional object in the interviews

Qualities of transitional object	Hank	Anthony	Holly	Anita	Cooper	Emerald	Abyss	Samuel
1 Assumes rights				✓				
2 Loved and mutilated	✓		✓					✓
3 Remains unchanged		✓	✓	✓	✓			✓
4 Survive loving and hating	✓		✓					✓
5 Vitality or reality of its own	✓	✓	✓	✓	✓	✓	✓	✓
6 Comes from within or without	✓	✓	✓	✓	✓	✓	✓	✓
7 Gradually de-cathected								

Note: ✓ represents the presence of the specific quality of the cigarettes in the interviews

We will examine each of the seven special qualities of the transitional object as outlined by Winnicott and discuss how these are manifested in the smoking behaviours, both from our own observations of smokers in the numerous qualitative focus group discussions and consumer interviews we have attended in the past 22 years with a global tobacco company, as well as from 16 interviews we conducted personally with eight respondents for the purpose of this book. Not all seven qualities are found in the interviews, and this could be due to first, the very open nature of the FANI method in which the content of the interviews is shaped by the respondents, hence some might prefer to cover more of the important events in their personal lives, rather than every single aspect of their smoking behaviours; and second, the limited time allocated for each interview, hence not all the respondents managed to cover all aspects of their smoking behaviours.

In the following section, we will be providing relevant snippets of the respondents' verbatim statements as they describe these emotionally charged smoking moments.

The first key transitional object quality as manifested consistently in the interviews: a cigarette is seen as more than merely a lifeless consumable object, but an object that has a life of its own

> 'Yet it must seem to the infant to give warmth, or to move, or to have texture, or to do something that seems to show it has vitality or reality of its own.'
>
> (Winnicott, 1953, p. 91)

Winnicott mentions four key components contributing to the transitional object being perceived as having a life of its own: it must be perceived as giving warmth, or to move, or to have texture, or to be doing something by itself. A cigarette and its consumption satisfy all the above componnents: by the time the cigarette smoke hits the smoker's lips, its temperature will have dropped from 400 to 900 degrees Celsius between puffs at the burning tip of the cigarette, to around 40 degrees Celsius at the mouth end of the filter, giving the smoker a warm sensation in their mouth, throat and lungs. Moreover, an entire smoking ritual is involved when people smoke; there is movement in the hands to light the cigarette, hold the cigarette towards their mouth while inhaling, and flicking ash between puffs. The entire smoking process involves fluid movement of the smoke while being drawn into the mouth and lungs during inhalation, circulating in the lungs and then removed from the body and mouth via exhalation of the smoke. It also involves a visual component as the stick gradually shortens with each puff of smoke from the cigarette; there is a visual burning zone at the tip of the cigarette and a building up of white ash on the, leaving only the cigarette stub when it is finished. These features add to the perception of the cigarette having a life of its own. This special quality of the transitional object appeared consistently in all the eight respondents' interviews, as is evident in the following extracts from their interview transcripts.

Hank's interviews

A cigarette is not just a cigarette, it is equivalent to a person in Hank's world, and smoking is like getting to know and build a relationship with that person. With the bad experience of his girlfriend cheating on him with his best friend, Hank seems to have lost a lot of faith in people. Sometimes he would rather not light his cigarettes, so he can preserve its life longer, and just like friendship which will eventually end, each cigarette will eventually get burnt out and 'die'.

> ... smoking a cigarette is like knowing a person ... there is an end to it, this relationship will end ... like when you know someone, that means it will end ... the relationship will eventually end ... I'd rather not know that person at all ... yeah, I don't even need to light the cigarette ...

> (Hank, second interview)

Anthony's interviews

Anthony struggled to verbalise what the cigarette represented in his life: its role changed from being a 'partner' who accompanies him when he is unhappy, to being just another 'hobby' to accompany him and it is a 'useful object' that he can rely on to do things. The description suddenly changed into 'animals' like cats and dogs, and finally it turned into a person like a 'friend', but perhaps not a very good friend, and it was afterwards downgraded to a 'pet' because he only plays with it when he needs it. Anthony mentioned very little about his mother during the interviews, or his family in general, and one wonders if the above contradictions depict his feelings towards his mother.

> ... I want to smoke when I am unhappy ... I feel like there is a partner with me when I smoke, yeah, it's like when you are unhappy, as a non-smoker you would weep sitting by the waterfront, but as a smoker like me, I would smoke a cigarette and weep sitting by the waterfront.

> (Anthony, first interview)

> ... so that a (smoking) moment is like another hobby to accompany you, it's not a human, I mean you can't describe it as having a life or soul, yeah, but it's an object, yeah! Something you can use to do things, something you can rely upon ... if it's not a person, perhaps it is an animal, yes! Like those cats and dogs, your pets ... it's very difficult to describe what it is, it is like a partner, or friend, but maybe not a very good friend ... it's more like an animal than a person, it's

not as important as a person … like a pet, you only play with it when you need it, you wouldn't normally play with it when you have something else to do.

(Anthony, second interview)

Holly's interviews

Holly displayed an extreme hatred and disgust towards a wet filter, as not only did it burn her fingers, but was also perceived almost like a monstrous object that needed to be got rid of immediately:

> … I would just put it (the filter) between my lips, and the filter wouldn't touch the wet part inside my mouth! … I mean once it's wet and after you've smoked it, the entire filter would turn yellow! … It gets really yellow when it's wet, and it also becomes soft, I mean the entire filter will be extremely soft … but I feel extremely uncomfortable to touch a wet filter with my dry lips! And then when I think again, that is actually saliva, and then you just can't stand it anymore, it's just not good! … you feel really hot when you suck in the smoke, I mean when the filter is flattened … it just burns your fingers … because you are holding the cigarette with your fingers. You can feel that it's really hot when you are holding that cigarette, it's really, really hot … if the filter is flattened. And also, it's really disgusting, the entire cigarette is deformed, I feel really disgusted and I don't like it! … Ah, I feel that it's really disgusting! It's unacceptable to me! I mean I really don't like the filter to be soaking wet!

(Holly, first interview)

Anita's interviews

The drawn in cigarette smoke was seen as being able to take away all the bad things from Anita, such as fatigue and grudges from customers. To Anita, a bad smoke is like troops of monsters made of newspapers and wastepaper rushing down her throat.

> … when I sat down and lit the cigarette, I sighed, I blew the smoke out, like blowing out all the fatigue, the grudges from customers, all were expelled …

(Anita, first interview)

What should a good (cigarette) taste like? When you smoke it, it should be so smooth, so slippery that it wouldn't choke your throat, you can draw it in smoothly. For cigarettes with a foul taste, you feel lots of impurities there when you draw it in, many strange things there, the smell would be very strange, you can't swallow it, you really can't draw it in, and you want to blow it out immediately. There is no way you can smoke another one, but there are no other choices, so I had to smoke that … I do feel lots of monsters in my throat. Before, people said they used newspapers and wastepaper to make the China flag [smuggled] cigarettes, so when I smoke those China flag cigarettes, I thought of many newspapers and wastepaper in my throat.

(Anita, first interview)

Cooper's interviews

A cigarette is equivalent to food for Cooper's mind and is seen as someone who is there and will always be there whenever they are needed, during good times and bad times.

[A cigarette] keeps me company when I am alone. It helps me when I am unhappy, happy, or when I've had a full meal. It's around all these times, it helps me whenever I need it ... Oh yes, happy and unhappy, I will smoke, I keep smoking. Its role is to stand by me whenever I have quarrels with my folks, or break up with my boyfriend, or go out drinking with my colleagues, in all these occasions, it is always next to me ... It is food to my mind ... I think it is feeding the need of my mind.

(Cooper, second interview)

Emerald's interviews

The inhaled smoke of the cigarette seems to have a life of its own and is able to circulate inside Emerald's body, including her lungs and brain. She finds it confusing as it is able to both destroy her, yet comfort and stimulate her.

... when I start smoking the cigarette on a normal day, it feels like it is injected into and then circling around my lungs, and then it comes out again, so my lungs would be inflated, the bone would be inflated! And then ... I would feel very confused, I would think that I am going to die, my lungs are getting darker and darker, and the smoke that is injected into my lungs is really strong ... and then I blow it out. On the other hand, it's really stimulating ... a big cloud of smoke getting inside, it's really comfortable, and then it comes out again ... just like that ... sometimes when I am in a rush, I would draw in a bigger puff ... if I want it to feel stronger, I just hold it and wait for it to get to my brain, to go around in my body, and then blow it out!

(Emerald, first interview)

Emerald also personified the inhaled and exhaled smoke as a person of the opposite sex who is highly unpredictable and changeable, who can fall passionately in love with you at one moment and leave you mercilessly at another, and all that can happen within a very short period of time.

... it (inhaled smoke) is like a person of the opposite sex, he is interested in you and you've just known him for a short while, and then he falls passionately in love with you, the emotion is very strong, the feeling that he gives you is very strong, very sweet and very happy. And then only after a short while, he suddenly leaves mercilessly ... after a short while, bye bye and he's blown out (exhaled smoke) ... it cools down immediately, cools down and drifts away!

(Emerald, first interview)

A cigarette is seen as Emerald's friend and soulmate who is always around and who has a life of their own; it is an ideal friend who knows exactly what she wants, and someone who is willing to devote all its life to her.

... a cigarette is my friend, yes, it is my friend! I mean when nobody understands me, it is the only one who understands me, it is at my beck and call. Whenever I am upset, it can always be lit whenever I find it, but I have to use money to buy it ... I would hide it when my family is around, but when I am with my friends then of course I don't mind, I would bring it out to meet my other real friends. Mmm ... we don't communicate, haha, but I feel that it would understand. I mean when I cry really hard, I don't really need to say anything, sometimes when I sing I would light a cigarette, and it would hear me, hahaha, yeah, so I feel that it's ... it's like my soulmate, we don't need to talk to each other but it knows what I am thinking about ... it's invisible, because it's my soulmate, it's my friend inside my heart and soul. It wouldn't come out to meet people unless it's necessary, I smoke by myself ... It won't be there under normal circumstances, but it will be there when I am very unhappy ... When my phone is gone, when there is nobody around me, I want to have a friend who wouldn't care about anything else but just sit beside me, and a cigarette is that friend ... A cigarette is like a friend who always sits beside me, it won't talk to me, but it lets me use it and helps me relax. I also feel that it's quite mighty, it won't talk back, and it won't criticise me, but it would let me ... I mean it devotes its whole life to me, lets me burn it all to ashes, in that sense it is really quite mighty.

(Emerald, second interview)

Abyss's interviews

Abyss saw cigarettes as mental food. While it hurts his throat he is still hopelessly addicted to this useless and harmful mental substance.

... I take it [cigarette] as my mental food, it's really like food ... it's like a mouthful of bad air getting in ... a mouthful of bad air. I know it's bad air, it sometimes tastes strong, I have a dry throat after excessive smoking ... everyone knows that it is a mouthful of bad air, but the demand is still there!

(Abyss, first Interview)

[a cigarette is like] a drug, yeah, as an analogy, and of course to me, stopping drugs is easier than stopping smoking ... I think stopping smoking is much more difficult than stopping drugs, right ... It [a cigarette] is something you draw in, something useless and harmful to you, so I can't find any analogy other than drugs.

(Abyss, second interview)

Samuel's interviews

Samuel is fascinated by the fluidity and changeability of the movement of cigarette smoke, and despite its malleability, Samuel also experiences its transient and fleeting nature.

So foggy, with clouds of smoke, so ... er ... the smoke and the fog, I feel the changes, it changes all the time like a kaleidoscope of shapes. You can play it in whatever form and shape you like. Like my friend is very good at blowing smoke circles, after drawing in the smoke, he blows out the smoke in the shape of circles. When many people smoke at the same time, the place gets foggy and it's covered in smoke, some people would write characters, or draw patterns in the smoke. Of course, it will disperse instantly, but they get to play with it first. I don't really play with the smoke. Yeah, but what kind of feeling I have with that? It changes all the time, you can play it in whatever form or shape you like, but it can't be touched, it is transient and fleeting, it disappears the moment it appears. This thing will disappear very quickly, it only stays there for a while, [seeing] the smoke rises up, or drifts off, and it's vanished, gone!

(Samuel, second interview)

The second key transitional object quality as manifested in the interviews: the location of the transitional object

'It comes from without from our point of view, but not so from the point of view of the baby. Neither does it come from within.'

(Winnicott, 1953, p. 91)

One unique characteristic of the complicated cigarette smoking process is that not only is the smoke inhaled by the lungs of the smoker, but the smoke also leaves the lungs through the exhalation process. The entire inhalation and exhalation process happens with each puff of smoke, consisting of seven puffs for each cigarette and an average daily consumption of eleven sticks per day for an average smoker. This movement between 'outside' and 'inside' happens 77 times each day during less than one hour per day's smoking time. Moreover, the smoke that is exhaled from the lungs is no longer the same smoke that is inhaled, because it was once 'merged' with the smoker when it entered his body, and 'separated' from the smoker after it left his body through exhalation. Hence, the exhaled smoke is no longer the same as the inhaled smoke because it has already passed through the smoker's body and hence was once part of the smoker. No other food product has similar characteristics of consumption, and this makes a cigarette a unique type of 'food' that has a special quality of frequent movement between what is external and what is internal, and the merging with and separating from the smoker from both a physical sensation and psychological perspective. This special quality of 'me' and 'not me', merging between the smokers and their cigarettes, appeared consistently in all eight respondents' interviews, as seen below.

Hank's interviews

Smoking seems to have taken Hank to a world that belongs entirely to him, this world gives him unspeakable comfort, a comfort that feels extremely relaxing. This magical world resembles the unchallenged transitional space described by Winnicott (1953). A cigarette can be seen as a very special form of an infantile transitional object in this unchallenged world, because it is not only an object, it is an object that requires the smokers to draw in the smoke to their body and blow it out to the environment, a state where 'me' (Hank) is merged with the 'not me' (the cigarette smoke). In phantasy, the consumption of a cigarette has a remarkable similarity to the infant sucking the mother's breast for milk and at the same time breathing out (projecting) their unspeakable anxieties to the mother (environment):

> … I feel that smoking is an enjoyment … How to say it … I mean it's like today I had lunch by myself, in Tsimshatsui East, I ate in an outdoor environment, I had a cigarette and some drinks by myself, I felt very comfortable, I don't know how to express that feeling. I mean, I was very free, very … I mean the sun … the sun was beaming down on me … I mean when I smoked this cigarette, I felt really enjoyable …
>
> (Hank, first interview)

> I don't know how to say it, I am not sure if it's my own problem, I mean I normally wouldn't tell others about my unhappiness … smoking a cigarette makes me feel that nothing has happened, I mean it's like swallowing an 'air' of anger … I smoke immediately whenever I am wronged, I mean I smoke whenever I get angry …
>
> (Hank, first interview)

> … I don't know, maybe it's my family education and training, I don't normally tell others about my problems and difficulties, so I feel that … how to say it … it's like maybe I have become dependent on cigarettes … maybe when you exhale the smoke … it's like … I don't know how to say it, it's a feeling … it's like when you exhale and blow out the smoke, it feels like you just get everything you want to say off your chest in one go … mmm … it's like you

feel completely relieved after you finish the cigarette, and you feel that maybe you've overthought things … it feels like the smoke takes away everything in one go, things like pressure … yeah, you blow everything out after you inhale, and then nothing has ever happened, it's all gone like magic!

(Hank, second interview)

… [when I smoked my ideal cigarette earlier today] I felt like I was the only one who existed in this entire world … I didn't need to worry about what others were doing, it was when I listened to music through headphones, and then I ate lunch by myself, so that world … at that time it completely belonged to me. It was also a very quiet world, I was the only one left in this world … [the cigarette] didn't really have a specific role in that world, it was a pure enjoyment, like when you are holding a wine glass … or when I play the guitar … you feel like you are the only one left in this world.

(Hank, second interview)

Anthony's interviews

To Anthony, smoking is the equivalent of breathing, an act that requires him to draw in the smoke to his lungs and exhale through his nose or mouth – pointing to a clear process of merging of the 'me' (Anthony) and the 'not me' (cigarette smoke). The inhalation of mentholated smoke from a menthol cigarette gives him a cooling sensation around his throat, and the exhalation gives him another wave of intense sensation, and only after he has experienced this intense sensation can he qualify as 'smoking for real.'

I've tried it [smoking a cigar] before, but I don't know what to do with it, because you tend to inhale the smoke into your lungs if you are used to smoking cigarettes, but if I just suck it in my mouth and I can't really talk, what do I do with it if I can't inhale it into my lungs? … I don't understand the kind of enjoyment people get by sucking and shaking it in your mouth [without inhaling it into your body] … if you only suck the smoke into your mouth without inhaling it into your lungs … what's the purpose of doing that? You are just holding some gas in your mouth, I mean would you hold the air in your mouth when you breathe? If you do that, your mouth wouldn't be comfortable, and you also can't speak! … I feel that it's a complete process only when you inhale it into your lungs, because if you don't inhale, you … you simply … don't know how it tastes like! If you don't get it down to this position [points to the level of his lung] … it doesn't get down, only your tongue would have the cigarette taste, and you also won't have that cooling sensation, the cooling sensation around that area when you smoke menthol cigarettes … I don't feel [the cooling sensation] much in my lungs, only around the throat area, and there is another wave of sensation when you exhale … after you inhale, you can exhale via your nose or your mouth. Yeah, and then when you exhale, you smoke [for real] … because you have to exhale after inhaling, right? … and when you exhale, it's … it's very important, this process! … I mean you would … you would be able to taste it [the smoke]. If you exhale with your nose, then its taste is even stronger! … you will feel the taste of the cigarette … yes, there is taste when you exhale, and the taste is even stronger if you exhale via your nose …

(Anthony, second interview)

Holly's interviews

The relationship between Holly and her cigarette is one that is similar to romantic love, a feeling that is very novel to her, a feeling that blurs the boundary between what's inside and outside as she becomes inseparable from her cigarettes, as if a pair of lovers become more inseparable as the love deepens over time. She loves to have her cigarette around, she loves to see it, she loves to eat [smoke] it, and she feels extremely unsettled and agitated whenever her cigarette is not around.

… but I don't smoke because of that [dizzy] feeling, I mean I really don't know why I am unable to separate myself from it! … Eh … huh … what … I don't know how to describe it! But I feel that eh … I know that I want this thing [a cigarette], not because I am addicted to it, but it's purely because I feel that I really love it, I love to see it and I love to eat (smoke) it. I mean it's not a matter of whether I need it or not, it's love! … in short, it's like I have this habit … So, I feel that I've always had this habit with me … my heart would convulse and beat faster if I don't have my cigarette, and then once I have it back I would feel … so comfortable! I just want this thing (a cigarette), so when I have it I would feel very comfortable. It's just like that, it's a real feeling you know?

(Holly, first interview)

… I mean, well, I used to only want to smoke a cigarette, but now when I smoke I feel like … eh … because I have never thought of my feelings towards cigarettes is equivalent to love, and then I feel like I love my cigarettes! I mean that feeling is very novel to me, yeah … that kind of love … like when you want to do something because you love doing that, but because of whatever reason you can't do it, then you feel unsettled and agitated … in short, it's not that I can't live without it, but … eh … it would be much better if I have it near me all the time. I mean, I would feel more comfortable that way, more settled, no matter what, I just feel that I need it [a cigarette] around!

(Holly, second interview)

Anita's interviews

To Anita, the smoking process makes the smell of the cigarette blend into her hands and her body, and when that happens the smell of the cigarette becomes the smell of her hands and her body. This familiar double experience gives her a feeling of intimacy with her Indonesian godfather whom she loves deeply, and an illusion of her still being together with him, which in turn provides her with a sense of security. Metaphorically, smoking feels like drawing in all the negative energy from the environment and using her own body to separate the bad from the good; the bad things get blown out from her body, leaving all the good things inside, so the good part of the drawn-in cigarette smoke merges with Anita in the smoking process.

> ... smoking is not about whether the taste is good or bad, it makes you feel at ease ... so smoking is like sitting on a massage chair, so comfortable. So ... a cigarette is an indispensable item ... The tobacco smell stays in the hand. Several hours after the smoke, you sniff your hand, it (the cigarette smell) gives you a feeling of intimacy ... smoking ... smelling the smoke gives me a sense of security! ... Smoking gives you a moment to rest, to think, to think things over, those things that are usually not thought of ... so I bought one stick (of my Indonesian dad's clove cigarette), and burned it, then smelled it ... I want to get that smell, that smell is the source of my sense of security, it helps me recollect how much he was fond of me when I was little, the time he was holding me in his arms, that sense of security feels so good. I want to feel it again through the [cigarette's] smell ...
>
> (Anita, first interview)

> ... like when you draw in (the smoke), it is like you suck in all the negative energy. Being in the world, sometimes you cannot speak your mind, something unhappy, you won't say it out loud, you let it stay inside your mouth. So when you draw in the smoke, you suck in the unhappy stuff which you want to say out loud but you cannot. Then you wait for it to be filtered, so the good stuff can be sucked in, the bad stuff gets blown out. What I blow out is what I don't like. Those blown out ... to the air, vanish in the air, it's pointless to think too much of it. Every issue needs a solution. So once you find the solution, it will be so nice. So smoking is a kind of a concept that there is always a way, a solution. If (the issue is) not solved, it will get stuck, and I won't be happy. So I must have a solution, (I must) force myself for this ... those that can't be comprehended, can't be understood and can't be solved, I just blow them all out ...'
>
> (Anita, second interview)

Cooper's interviews

Cooper established a strong link between smoking and her emotions. In her phantasy, she is always alone when she smokes in this space; the cigarette smoke becomes a part of her and it merges with her body when she draws it in. The smoke also helps absorb all the badness and unhappiness in moments when she is sad, for example, after breaking up with her boyfriend, the bad emotions will be expelled from her completely when she blows out the cigarette smoke. This is a strong indication of the smoke merging with Cooper as one, and its function which is to take away all the badness from Cooper and project it onto the environment.

> … when I was unhappy, like after breaking up with my boyfriend, I just smoked, smoked, and smoked, and then blew the smoke out. Afterwards I just cried, cried and cried. I felt like … how should I put it … maybe there is only me in the world [of smoking] … I really don't know how to express it, probably just want to blow it [the smoke] all out, then all would be gone, out! I think smoking and emotions are closely linked together …
>
> (Cooper, first interview)

Emerald's interviews

Emerald vividly described the world of smoking as equivalent to a resting place, a place where she could detach herself from the outside world for a brief moment in a separated and yet connected place, as seen in the transparent protective shield analogy used by Emerald to describe the connectedness and yet separateness of the two worlds. In this world that is connected and yet separated from the real world, Emerald can sink in completely (merging of 'me' and 'not me') and enjoy a moment of quietness and peace before returning to the real world.

> … I mean I feel like I can take a rest there (when I smoke), but I need to go back after I finish the smoke … I only went there to take a rest, mmm … and after taking a rest I will need to … eh … do whatever I need to do afterwards. So, it [smoking] gives me a moment of quietness and peace … [this world of smoking is connected and yet separated by] a transparent protective shield (from the real world) …'
>
> (Emerald, second interview)

Abyss's interviews

The world that smoking can transport him to is a world that is hidden under his blanket in his bed, somewhere he can wriggle in or crawl under, somewhere that does not have any contact with the outside world. This secret world seems to resemble a regression towards an inter-uterine life. In Abyss's phantasy world, smoking a cigarette brings him back to the womb of his mother, a place where Abyss is buried in his mother's body and therefore does not have any contact with the real world, a place where he can once again merge with his mother where the 'me' and 'not me' experience becomes blurred. Abyss crawls in deeper and deeper as the sense of insecurity increases in the real world, as manifested by him drawing in more and more smoke in.

> … that world [with the most disappointing cigarette] is none of my business anymore, I just wanted to leave, don't think [anymore], just jump over it … I

wanted to find a hole to wiggle in, yeah, wanted to find a hole to wiggle in …
there was no sense of security, I felt insecure at that time, just wanted to find a
hole to wiggle in, or crawl under my blanket in bed. So, in a word, just don't let
me have any contact with the [outside] world … [the drawn in smoke] made me
feel decadent, feel sorry for myself … decadent … that made me feel so insecure. Just like suddenly shut down from the outside world. Yeah, so I drew one
more puff, I knew that it wouldn't give me any particular sensation [satisfac-
tion], anyway, I just couldn't think of anything at that moment, I was so scared
and insecure, I just didn't want to be in contact with the outside world.'

(Abyss, second interview)

Samuel's interviews

Smoking can take Samuel to an ideal, dream-like world that is purely enjoyable, a
world where he doesn't have to think about what's happening outside, a world that
belongs solely to him and that he can be fully immersed in, and a world where he
can feel content. This world is partly detached from and yet partly connected to the
real world: partly detached because there is no one else apart from Samuel in that
world, partly connected because Samuel is conscious that he will need to go back to
the real world after a few minutes of pure indulgence and enjoyment in this dream-
like world. To Samuel, a cigarette is something that exists in both the real world
and the ideal, dream-like world; it is something that makes the ideal, dream-like
world perfect: it is both an object that can transport Samuel to the ideal, dream-like
world, as well as an object that takes him back to the real world, when the cigarette
is smoked out. In the dream-like world, the cigarette ['not me'] is merged with
Samuel ['me'] as one unit as he travels in the space between the two worlds.

> … the ideal cigarette I had was yesterday in Stanley. I was with my girlfriend
> in Stanley. Unlike me, she doesn't smoke. So, I stole a chance, told her that I
> wanted to go to the toilet, and in fact I went to smoke instead. Sitting by the sea-
> side watching the sunset, this is what one calls 'truly enjoyable!' … I felt very
> content. The world was purely wonderful during those few minutes. The feeling
> was gone when I finished the smoke, and I had to go back again … returning
> to the real world again … I love smoking in a comfy environment. When I'm
> watching the open sea, it gives me a feeling of calmness, very comfy … I don't
> like being hectic, I like the comfy feeling, I like to feel free, so … maybe it's
> because of my personality, I would feel content as long as the environment can
> give me a sense of comfort and relaxation … so I would feel peaceful even when
> I am standing next to a trash bin while I am smoking!'
>   … if there is no one at home, I enjoy sitting in the living room quietly smok-
> ing my cigarette … do nothing, think of nothing, no need to use my brain, time
> seems to have stopped. That moment belongs to me completely, and I have to
> return to the real world again a few minutes after I finish smoking … so it's that
> feeling … which is not easy to describe … I like smoking in a comfy environ-
> ment, not necessarily beautiful, but comfy, with no one there to both me, as

simple as that … (In there, time) stopped for a short while … (I guess) I would still feel comfy even without a cigarette in that quiet environment, but something is missing, that's what a cigarette can give me … with a cigarette there (in that quiet and comfy space), the world becomes perfect! … it (a cigarette) is kind of soft, a cigarette makes me feel soft, gives me a sense of peacefulness, it belongs to the quiet type … liquor, on the contrary, is very masculine and heroic. The ambiance I like is the quiet type, so I need something soft to go with me, then I will feel satisfied … a cigarette belongs to the real world, but I'd love to take my cigarette to the other (ideal, dream-like) world, and when the cigarette is smoked out, I know it's time to return to reality!

(Samuel, second interview)

Other transitional object qualities manifested in the different stages of interviews amongst the eight respondents

'The infant assumes rights over the object …'

(Winnicott, 1953, p. 91)

The strong sense of ownership of their cigarettes can be seen in the following transcript from Cooper and Anita:

I have a god-brother, we are very close. We were very poor when we first met, the whole gang was penniless, no job, but we still went out for fun, to an extent we only had a few pennies left for the bus, then we rallied for money. At that time, it was HK$29 a packet (of cigarettes). After fund rallying, we just got enough to buy one packet. Well there weren't enough cigarettes to split among so many of us, so we could only take it by puffs. And sometimes, some people just took away the cigarette without returning it to the group. So, when I was smoking, I was so afraid that he would just take it away, so I just held the cigarette for him to draw in, and then he would suddenly turn away and take the cigarette away in his mouth! … I was really angry then, because I was really penniless, and I didn't have enough cigarettes for myself!

(Cooper, second interview)

No, it [the cigarette] won't [leave me]. At most, you leave cigarettes. They won't leave me for no reason … Cigarettes have a lower status than workers. Of course, the partner comes first. Only a minor difference between the partner and workers. Because you can own the partner, but you can't own the workers … you can own cigarettes, but cigarettes can also affect others …

(Anita, first interview)

'The object is affectionately cuddled as well as excitedly loved and mutilated.'

(Winnicott, 1953, p. 91)

'It must survive instinctual loving, and also hating ...'

(Winnicott, 1953, p. 91)

A global, principal product developer of a multinational tobacco company once mentioned at a conference that 'the relationship between the smokers and the cigarettes is very personal, people kiss (smoke) this product ten to twelves times a day (ten to twelve sticks per day) and six to seven kisses each time (six to seven puffs for each stick of cigarette) ... you kiss the cigarettes more than your wife ... you drink cigarettes every day!' The above quotation illustrates the intimate loving relationship between smokers and their cigarettes; the smokers kiss and drink the cigarettes multiple times a day, an act that is a lot more intimate than cuddling. This is a very interesting coincidence with respect to the famous quote by Freud in his letter to his fiancée, Martha Bernays, during the time when he was very preoccupied with all the kisses he could not give her because of the distance between them. In one letter dated 22 January 1884, Freud attributed his addiction to cigars to her absence and said, 'smoking is indispensable if one has nothing to kiss' (Gay, 1988, p. 39). The following verbatim transcription of the interviews illustrates how the respondents demonstrated their love towards their cigarettes.

Hank dropped into a world of his own when he talked about how beautiful his empty cigarette pack collection was, as if he was describing a piece of art created by him. The emotion displayed by Hank on his 'cigarette art' could be seen as an indication of the object being affectionately cuddled and excitedly loved:

> ... I collect empty cigarette packs! Yes, empty packs, I arranged them all in the room, in the cabinet, they are very beautiful! ... I only started doing that in the past six months ... so beautiful, I think ... they all lined up together in a row, very beautiful!"

(Hank, first interview)

A strong desire of love for her cigarettes was seen when Holly talked about how much she is unable to separate herself from them:

> I don't smoke because of that (dizzy) feeling, I mean I really don't know why I am unable to separate myself from it! ... I don't know how to describe it! But I feel that eh ... I know that I want this thing [a cigarette], not because I am addicted to it, but it's purely because I feel that I really love it, I love to see it and I love to eat [smoke] it. I mean it's not a matter of whether I need it or not, it's love!

(Holly, first interview)

... my heart would convulse and beat faster if I don't have my cigarette, and then once I have it back I would feel ... so comfortable! I just want this thing [a cigarette], so when I have it I would feel very comfortable. It's just like that, it's a real feeling you know?

(Holly, first interview)

... when I smoke I feel like ... eh ... because I have never thought of my feelings towards cigarettes is equivalent to love, and then I feel like I love my cigarettes! I mean that feeling is very novel to me, yeah, like ... that kind of love ... eh ... in fact it's like ... it's like you love .... I won't say it's a habit, but habit is also driven by love, and that's why you have this habit to start with!

(Holly, second interview)

Instinctual love of his cigarette is seen in the insatiable hunger that is triggered when Abyss smokes:

Everything, every single incident ... when it happens, there is always a beginning and an end .... once you've reached the end you would feel satisfied. But smoking is not like that. I desire to smoke, but when I finish smoking, I would smoke a second one, a third one, a fourth one, a fifth one. So, smoking will never fulfil the desire for satisfaction. It won't ... unless smoking can give me a great sense of success ... I think smoking could give me satisfaction only under one condition, when I stop smoking! Right, if I want to get satisfaction from smoking, I probably need to take this step, and stop smoking!

(Abyss, second interview)

The love for the cigarette is seen in Samuel's enjoyment of it as being equivalent to a 'full feed':

... [my ideal cigarette is] the cigarette after a full meal ... yesterday ... we usually smoke after we feed our stomach, so the feeling is "full", very satisfying. A bit drowsy after the meal, in full stomach, smoking makes us feel soothed, very relaxed, so comfy after the full meal, so full, in this sleepiness, smoking a cigarette makes me feel soothed and satisfied ... the cigarette after a full meal is so relaxing, I smoke slowly, very slowly ... the cigarette after a meal is a slow smoking [moment], savouring it ... I feel very relaxed, comfy.

(Samuel, first interview)

On the other hand, when a smoker smokes his cigarette, the cigarette is shortened during the consumption process, but it is never completely destroyed, for there is always a cigarette stub remaining. Therefore, symbolically, it resembles the cigarette being mutilated (shortened) and yet surviving the attack (the remaining cigarette stub). Another obvious sign of mutilation of the cigarette is the filter-biting behaviour which is very common in countries like South Korea and Japan. Hank's filter biting could be seen as an act of mutilation and the cigarette survives his hate:

> ... I didn't feel it myself, but I have a habit of biting the filter ... which means my cigarette filter will be all wet after I smoke it, and I would bite it and hold it in my mouth after I finish smoking it ... I mean I just bite it while I smoke ... it's easier to suck if you bite it ...
>
> (Hank, first interview)

> ... sometimes the filter would fall off ... just throw the cigarette away! ... can't smoke it anymore, I mean the filter becomes very soft and wet after I have bitten it ... and then I just throw the cigarette away!
>
> (Hank, second interview)

> ... when my friends ask me to share my cigarette with them, they would im-mediately know that the cigarette is mine because my filter would always be flat and wet, yeah, I only realised that I have this filter biting habit when my friends told me about it, I didn't know everybody else did not bite the filter! ... do you understand what I am talking about? ... because I feel that there is no taste if you just smoke the cigarette without biting the filter, the filter will become firmer when you bite it, and you can inhale more, such a wonderful experience!
>
> (Hank, second interview)

Instinctual hating of the most disappointing cigarette by Holly can be seen below:

> ... I suppose it didn't satisfy my need ... I felt that 'wow, this cannot satisfy my needs at all!' Completely not what I wanted! Then I felt that this cigarette was really unstable, and that all Capri Superslims cigarettes are 'unstable!' Anyway, it means it didn't satisfy my needs at all, it failed completely! ... It's not good enough. I feel that it's totally bad!
>
> (Holly, second interview)

> 'It must never be changed, unless changed by the infant'
>
> (Winnicott, 1953, p. 91)

Out of all other fast-moving consumer goods, the cigarette is probably the one single product that has not changed much over the past century: a cigarette today still pretty much looks the same as the first machine-made commercial cigarette of 1881. Major innovations in the tobacco industry include the introduction of the perceived to be 'safer' filtered cigarettes by the 1960s, after the U.S. Surgeon Gen-eral linked smoking to lung cancer in 1964. Apart from the filter, there are varying levels of tar in cigarettes, slightly different lengths and circumferences, while others have different filter shapes. Some manufacturers add different flavours to the cigarette using different technologies. There have been numerous attempts by the tobacco industry to introduce new innovations in the market in the past century, but very few are accepted by consumers. Generally speaking, smokers are highly resistant to change, both in terms of the cigarette brands they smoke as well as the actual product itself. For instance, tobacco brands enjoy a higher than 90 per cent loyalty level, which means that more than 90 per cent of smokers have already decided which brand to purchase when they enter a shop, and there is little anyone can do to change their mind. Moreover, there have been a number of classic case studies undertaken by the tobacco industry where a small change in the filter design provoked a sharp drop in market share, indicating an extreme reaction by smokers to the slightest change in design, who were convinced that the product taste had also been changed. Such extreme reactions are evidenced in the following transcripts.

Anthony believed that all the changes to his cigarettes in the past made them taste worse and he did not like any of these changes. Marlboro Black was the first cigarette brand he used to smoke regularly, and he believed that its taste had got stronger and stronger. In reality, cigarettes usually contain lower rather than higher tar as time goes by, driven partly by government imposed regulations on tar levels and partly by a natural smoking progression from high to low tar. So, the following account could only be a perception rather than a reality:

> There was this Marlboro Black, its packaging was in black and green colour, I used to smoke it regularly, my classmates also bought it all the time, but now … really … I wouldn't smoke it even if it was free! … because I felt that the taste is different … maybe they changed the taste after market research! … I used to think that Marlboro Black was really tasty, and gradually I felt that … oh, how come it seems to taste more and more disgusting? And then … yeah, I just stopped smoking it! … Because it used to taste quite mild, and then I felt that the smoke smelt worse every day, like it's penetrated into your body, you feel like an old and seriously addicted chain smoker after smoking it! … your whole body is contaminated by that smell, and it never goes away! So, I didn't want to smoke it anymore after finishing one stick, and I could still smell the bad taste even after walking outside for a long time!
>
> (Anthony, second interview)

To Anthony, any change to his cigarette is equivalent to a deterioration of its quality, so, only the original is best, and no change is tolerated.

> Good [quality of cigarettes] means … the taste is the same as the first time I smoked it!
>
> (Anthony, second interview)

Cooper's held an irrational belief that Marlboro Ice Blue's taste had changed:

> ... Marlboro Ice Blue, it has changed! All of a sudden it tastes differently! No matter where I buy it, I just feel that it tastes differently! I don't know what exactly the difference is, anyway, the taste is just different! ... I wondered if it is a counterfeit, because I am concerned with what stuff they put in there ... once I realise the difference in taste, it makes me nervous, not sure if it is a counterfeit, I don't know what stuff they've added to the cigarettes! ... but I even bought it in 7–11, there is no way that 7–11 would sell counterfeit cigarettes! ... Yes, I did [get very angry]. I stopped smoking it for one, two packs, but I smoked it again afterwards as its taste just miraculously came back ... despite the anger ... maybe it has not changed at all!
>
> (Cooper, first interview)

Holly expresses her disgust when a cigarette is 'changed' by having a deformed and wet filter:

> ... it's a piece of cotton, right? I mean once it's wet and after you've smoked it, the entire filter would turn yellow! ... you feel really hot when you suck in the smoke, I mean when the filter is flattened ... it just burns your hand! ... you can feel that it's really hot when you are holding that cigarette, it's really, really, hot ... if the filter is flattened. And also, it's really disgusting, the entire cigarette is deformed, I feel really disgusted and I don't like it!
>
> (Holly, first interview)

Samuel was enraged when he talked about the change of price (due to government excise increase), the change of the form (due to rain), and the change of mind of the manufacturer of his cigarettes (due to cessation of production):

> ... it's not fair! Tax on red wine and cigars is reduced but increases on cigarettes! But red wine and cigars are for rich people, and cigarettes are for commoners ... commoners smoke cigarettes and drink beer. But those items used by the upper class got reduced (tax), and the commoners' increased. It makes me angry! ... I will get angry; I feel that it's not fair. Why did you reduce excise on red wine and cigars? If you want to increase excise, increase it on all of them, you can't be that partial! ... because it is not the first time. When they increased it [the cigarette price] from $29 to $39, there was a reduction on red wine! When it was increased to $55, tax reduction continued on red wine! I didn't mind it much when it was increased from the twenties to thirties, it might only be just that time, but you did it time and again! You are doing it on purpose!
>
> (Samuel, first interview)

> My cigarette was soaked in rain! ... (after a whole day of meaningless open day programme at school) once the recess came, I ran out to smoke in no time, to

relax, to get comfy. I lit the cigarette, then came the rain! The whole stick got soaked in rain! ... the rain just came down on me before I finished drawing the first puff! The whole stick was completely wet. No more smoking. I was wet too, then I went back in ... I just wanted to smoke, why on earth did they do that to me! That's how I felt (furious)! Afterwards, I walked back in to borrow an umbrella from someone, and I smoked while holding the umbrella! ... I didn't want it to end (finish) like that! I lit the cigarette and I was not done with it yet, and it ended! So, I smoked the second one to compensate for that! ... when it's pouring rain, the cigarette easily gets soaking wet, and it breaks apart, then I am really angry!

(Samuel, second interview)

Winfield menthol was my first cigarette ... the taste was very minty, like eating mint candies. Then they stopped producing them. Then I got so angry for a period of time! ... very angry, because they stopped producing them, they were irreplaceable! It was my first encounter of this thing (smoking). I might change to another taste (cigarette) later, god knows, but I didn't want to at that point in time, I kind of felt like 'why are you forcing me to change?' ... I was much angrier about Winfield (being discontinued, compared to his cigarette being soaked in rain)! ... I was so angry that I wanted to blow Winfield's office into pieces! ... that time when I began to look for my cigarettes and found that they were out of stock. I didn't pay much attention to it at first, because I thought they were only temporarily out of stock ... afterwards, I kept looking for them, and one day, they just stopped producing them completely, no production, no stock! So, they were not out of stock! So, no stock because no production, then I got furious!

(Samuel, second interview)

Its fate is to be gradually allowed to be decathected, so that in the course of years it becomes not so much forgotten as relegated to limbo ...'

(Winnicott, 1953, p. 91)

In Cooper's everyday life, the cigarette is forgotten and taken for granted when she is happy and enjoying her time with her friends, so the cigarette is like a loyal companion to Cooper, there to comfort her only when she is unhappy.

... when you are happy, you won't stop to smoke. However, it takes about five minutes to smoke a cigarette – it is impossible to sit still for five minutes to finish that cigarette. You look around at the people around you, and you are compelled to join them. Therefore, I would smoke only a little of the cigarette, perhaps just half of it, then stub it out and join the group. Then afterwards, when

I crave for a smoke, I would just get another one and the process repeats. On the other hand, when I am unhappy, the cigarette is like a companion keeping me company and I don't want to waste it. It is the only thing there for me and so I will focus on it and won't leave it aside.

(Cooper, second interview)

Part VI

So what?

In previous chapters, we explored the literature and research related to smoking addiction from the perspectives of academic psychology, psychoanalysis and the tobacco industry; we have also deep-dived into Winnicott's idea of the transitional object in order to understand its value in the understanding of smoking addiction, and specifically, how a cigarette resembles the transitional object, as demonstrated in the 16 interview transcripts gathered from eight smokers, in line with Winnicott (1953).

Now that we have established the main argument for the book, that a cigarette can be regarded as a regressed form of infantile transitional object that re-appears in adulthood, we will be considering the implications of this conclusion in terms of what it means for smokers and public health policy, as well as some proposed directions for future research.

Key sections

- Implications for smokers and public health policy
- Proposed directions for future research

Based on the results of our research, the smoking experience bears a close resemblance to the highly intense and private experience of the transitional space as described by Winnicott (1953). In this very special type of transitional space experienced by the smokers, the cigarette is consistently used as an instrument to facilitate immediate entry into the transitional space and thus, an intense experience.

The characteristic of this instrument (a cigarette) has a striking similarity to the infantile transitional object described by Winnicott: despite the limited time allocated to the interviews, two out of the seven special characteristics of the transitional object are consistently manifested in the respondents' interviews, that is, the object being perceived as having a life of its own, and the location of the object being in the intermediate area between internal and external reality. Given the results, I suggest that these two special qualities of transitional object are the most

DOI: 10.4324/9781003329077-23

definitive qualities that are able to differentiate a transitional object from a normal soothing object.

The idea of the reappearance of the transitional object in adulthood may sound paradoxical at first glance, because theoretically speaking the transitional object should only appear in infancy, as indicated by Winnicott:

> I suggest that the pattern of transitional phenomena begins to show at about 4–6–8–12 months … an infant's transitional object ordinarily becomes gradually decathected, especially as cultural interests develop.
>
> (Winnicott, 1953, p. 97)

However, it is also important to note that Winnicott also suggested in the same paper that there is a possibility for the reappearance of the infantile transitional object in adulthood when the person is threated by deprivation:

> Purposely I leave room for wide variations. Patterns set in infancy may persist into childhood, so that the original soft object continues to be absolutely necessary at bedtime or at time of loneliness or when a depressed mood threatens. In health, however, there is a gradual extension of range of interest, and eventually the extended range is maintained, even when depressive anxiety is near. A need for a specific object or a behaviour pattern that started at a very early date may reappear at a later age when deprivation threatens.
>
> (Winnicott, 1953, p. 91)

There is, therefore, a possibility for the reappearance of the need for the transitional object even in adulthood if threatened by deprivation, loneliness, or at night when one moves through sleep from the external world to the internal world.

Winnicott gave three examples in relation to the pathological development and reappearance of the transitional object in adulthood. In psychopathology:

> Addiction can be stated in terms of regression to the early stage at which the transitional phenomena are unchallenged;
>
> Fetish can be described in terms of a persistence of a specific object or type of object dating from infantile experience in the transitional field, linked with the delusion of a maternal phallus;
>
> Pseudologia and thieving can be described in terms of an individual's unconscious urge to bridge a gap in continuity of experience in respect of a transitional object.
>
> (Winnicott, 1953, p. 97)

Smoking addiction may be classified under the 'addiction' category of psychopathology: instead of following a healthy development path in which the transitional space is expanded over the entire cultural field and the transitional object is no longer needed, when threatened by deprivation, the smoker resorts to cigarettes that can transport him to an intermediate area, a resting place where he can re-experience a blissful infantile reunion while merging with his mother. This happens as soon as he lights up the cigarette and draws in the first puff of smoke, as if by magic. To the smoker, a cigarette functions as a regressed form of infantile transitional object that may help initiate this regressive experience on demand. This book provides evidence to support Winnicott's idea of the reappearance of transitional object in adulthood when a person is threatened by deprivation, an idea that Winnicott himself did not further elaborate on after mentioning it in the 1953 work.

Chapter 17

Implications for smokers and public health policy

Despite the known effect of nicotine on increasing levels of dopamine, the neurotransmitter that induces feelings of pleasure and reward, a smoking addiction involves much more than a pharmacological effect, otherwise nicotine replacement therapy would have already been a successful tool to help people stop smoking. The results of the current thesis further suggest that conscious and rational factors alone are unable to account for the irrational behaviours displayed by educated and intelligent people who continue to smoke despite understanding the risks of smoking. The unique physical characteristics and the consumption process of a cigarette make it capable of evoking highly primitive associations and memories in smokers. Even Sigmund Freud, the father of psychoanalysis, was unable to stop smoking despite multiple attempts in the span of 45 years. At one time, after stopping smoking for 14 months due to health reasons, Freud decided to resume smoking again, stating that he was unable to stop smoking cigars, and 'the torture being beyond human power to bear' (Jones, 1972, p. 341). Freud continued to smoke an average of 20 cigars a day until he died.

What is the kind of 'torture' that is 'beyond human power to bear'? If we go back to infancy, the origin of our lives, we may say that no torture is more severe than the torture of separation from one's mother, our first love object, someone who was equivalent to our entire world. Worst of all, from an infant's perspective, the separation is perceived as the death of the mother, no matter how short the duration is.

The resemblance of the relationship between the smoker and their cigarette, and the infant and its transitional object, renders cigarettes as a regressed form of transitional object *par excellence*. To the infant, the transitional object is its first possession, it is a part of itself like a mouth or a breast, and it is also a substitute for its mother and a representation of its omnipotence as the infant begins to bridge the subjective and objective experience and separate the 'me' from the 'not me'. Therefore, it is simply unimaginable for the infant to lose or discontinue its relationship with the transitional object at this stage of its development. By the same token, from a smoker's perspective, stopping smoking is similar to weaning, or getting an infant to cut off its relationship with the transitional object and letting go of the blissful reunion with one's mother, when one can rest and feel safe again, hence an infantile violent attack is inevitable. Therefore, the primitive experience evoked in

DOI: 10.4324/9781003329077-24

the entire smoking process is comparable to the kind of 'intense experiencing that belongs to the arts and to religion and to imaginative living, and to creative scientific work' (Winnicott, 1953, p. 97).

Taking this into consideration, from the smokers' perspective, it is important for them to be aware of the primitive nature of their smoking behaviour, and how it resembles a regressed form of transitional object that re-appears in adulthood. Once the smokers are made aware of the fact that the 'prize' that they repeatedly look for in smoking their cigarettes is not the taste of the cigarette nor the addictive nicotine content, but the 'intense experiencing' in the intermediate space resembling the blissful reunion with their mother and their infantile experience of omnipotence, they then can be exposed to other ways to achieve a similar 'intense experiencing', such as arts, religion, imaginative living and creative scientific work as suggested by Winnicott (1953). This insight will lead to a very different approach in helping smokers reduce their dependence on cigarettes.

Given the highly primitive nature of experience involved in the smoking process, and the unbearable torture that is 'beyond human power to bear', cigarettes as a category of product are here to stay because there will always be demand for them. From a government's perspective, instead of trying to reduce smoking incidence with tactics such as excise increases, flavour and ingredient ban, plain packaging, graphic health warnings or cigarette pack display bans, a more effective strategy would be to encourage the development of reduced harm products that resemble the physical characteristics of cigarettes, while at the same time retain the majority of the smoking rituals.

The recent development of vapour and tobacco heating products from the global tobacco companies is on the right track in getting smokers to move away from tobacco to less harmful alternatives, as these devices either do not contain tobacco and combustion, in the case of vapour, or they heat the tobacco to below combustion temperature and hence can stop the production of tar, the most harmful by-product of tobacco smoking. Having said that, both vapour and tobacco heating products deliver an inferior, though acceptable, smoking experience compared to traditional cigarettes, because they do not burn to the butts when consumed, as in the case of traditional cigarettes, so they lack the 'aliveness' quality of cigarettes (the fifth quality of the transitional object suggested by Winnicott).

Chapter 18

Proposed directions for future research

A longitudinal study to understand the impact of parents' child rearing practices on smoking addiction in adulthood

According to Winnicott, transitional phenomena and the transitional object are the basis of initiation of experience and object relations of the infant, hence signs of a healthy development that is made possible by the presence of a 'good enough mother', who, in a state of 'primary maternal preoccupation', continuously adapts to the needs of the infant by gradually introducing appropriate doses of external reality to it. This is done by creating a 'holding environment' and an illusion that reinforces the infant's feelings of omnipotence, an illusion that the infant is capable of creating an outer reality that could relieve instinctual tension, and that the breast is part of the infant's creation and is therefore under its magical control. If this illusion can be successfully established, a good internal object is created and the 'good enough mother' can start to gradually disillusion the infant by bringing small experiences of the world to it, as its capacity to tolerate frustration increases over time.

However, there is a group of 'not-good-enough mothers' who constantly fail to adapt to the needs of the infant, and they can be further divided into three types:

> The psychotic mother may well be able to cope with the small infant's demands in the beginning, but she is not able to be separated from the infant as it needs to grow away from her preoccupation. The mother who does not naturally find herself in a state of primary maternal preoccupation – perhaps because she is too depressed or preoccupied with something else – may later on have to be a therapist for her child, who is likely to be seeking compensation for the earlier loss. The tantalising mother has, for Winnicott, the worst effect on her infant's mental health, as the erratic nature of the environment violates the very core sense of self.
> (Abram, 2007, pp. 243–244)

These 'not-good-enough mothers' seduce the infant into developing a pathological, false compliant self to cope with their own maternal failure, resulting in the ego distortion of the infant, which is the basis of schizoid characteristics in adulthood; or it can result in the development of a self-holding defence mechanism in which a

DOI: 10.4324/9781003329077-25

caretaker false self is formed (Winnicott, 1956). Winnicott's view is consistent with Milner (1952), who suggests that maternal failure is a precursor to premature ego-development and a disturbed illusionary period. Because of this disturbance, the ego is forced into precocious differentiation between the bad and the good object, and the individual can go through life searching for the valuable 'resting place' of illusion that they missed in their early childhood.

If smoking addiction falls into the realm of regression to the infantile transitional phenomena, using Winnicott's (1953) concepts of the 'psychotic mother' who never weans the infant, an interesting question would be, to what extent the 'psychotogenic mother', that is, the mother who causes psychosis in her baby, contributes to the prolonged use of cigarettes by the smoker as a regressed transitional object in order to deal with separation anxiety and sustain their omnipotent delusion when confronted with deprivation?

Based on Winnicott's idea of the connection between addiction and regression to the infantile transitional phenomena in adulthood, as well as the 'psychotic mother' idea, we were at first also interested in exploring the relationship between a 'not-good-enough mother' and her child's smoking addiction in adulthood. However, in the absence of an available psychoanalytic research methodology to analyse the child-rearing practices of the smokers' mothers over 20 years ago, which would have provided understanding of the quality of mothering delivered at that time, it has proved to be almost impossible to investigate this part of our research question for this present work. This is also due to the fact that memory and recollection is prone to distortion and unreliability over time.

Future researchers are encouraged to conduct a longitudinal study involving both the respondents and their parents using direct observations over a period of at least 18 years, in order to understand the impact of the environment (the mother and the father) on the propensity of smoking addiction of the respondents.

Researching the entire smoking process including the breathing process related to smoking

The smoking process involves three different aspects: the cigarette is used as an instrument (transitional object) to help smokers enter the transitional space when they draw in and blow out the cigarette smoke. Therefore, there is the instrument (transitional object), the smoking moment (transitional phenomena), and the breathing related to the inhalation and exhalation of cigarette smoke.

The current study only focuses on the first two stages: the transitional object and the transitional phenomena related to smoking addiction. More understanding is needed on the breathing stage in terms of how it relates to and impacts the smoking experience and smoking addiction.

The formulation of a new smoking cessation approach?

If cigarettes can be regarded as a regressed form of transitional object that re-appear in adulthood, then the 'prize' that the smokers repeatedly look for by smoking cigarettes is the 'intense experiencing' or the intermediate space resembling the blissful reunion with the mother and the ensuing infantile experience of omnipotence. If this is correct, then it would be worthwhile considering the possibility of providing a method or instrument for smokers so that they might enter this transitional space with 'intense experiencing' through means other than cigarettes, for example, cultural experiences such as the arts, religion, imaginative living and creative scientific work (Winnicott, 1953). This would also mean that we would be creating smoking cessation programmes with a completely different approach.

There is very little research being conducted on smoking addiction outside of the tobacco industry itself, I hope this book will be a stimulus for more research into smoking addiction from academic research which is not funded by tobacco companies.

References

Abraham, K. (1926). The psychological relations between sexuality and alcoholism. *The International Journal of Psychoanalysis, 7*, 2.

Abram, J. (2007). *The language of Winnicott: a dictionary of Winnicott's use of words* (2nd ed.) Karnac Books.

Adler, G. (1989). Transitional phenomena, projective identification, and the essential ambiguity of the psychoanalytic situation. *The Psychoanalytic Quarterly, 58*(1), 81–104.

Adler, N. (1986). Sublimation and addiction: complementarities and antitheses. *Psychoanalytic Psychology, 3*(2), 187.

Agar, M., & Reisinger, H. S. (2002). A heroin epidemic at the intersection of histories: the 1960s epidemic among African Americans in Baltimore. *Medical Anthropology, 21*(2), 115–156.

Ainsworth, M. D., & Wittig, B. A. (1969). Attachment and exploratory behaviour of one-year-olds in a strange situation. In B. M. Foss (Ed.), *Determinants of infant behaviour VI* (pp. 113–136). Methuen.

Athanassiou, C. (1991). Construction of a transitional space in an infant twin girl. *International Review of Psychoanalysis, 18*, 53–63.

Audrain-McGovern, J., Rodriguez, D., Tercyak, K. P., Epstein, L. H., Goldman, P. & Wileyto, E. P. (2004). Applying a behavioural economic framework to understanding adolescent smoking. *Psychology of Addictive Behaviour, 18*(1), 64–73.

Azorlosa, J. L. (1994). The effect of chronic naltrexone pretreatment on associative vs. non-associative morphine tolerance. *Drug and Alcohol Dependence, 36*(1), 65–67.

Balfour, D. K. J. (2004). The neurobiology of tobacco dependence: a preclinical perspective on the role of the dopamine projections to the nucleus accumbens. *Nicotine and Tobacco Research, 6*(6), 899–912.

Bartos, R. (1977). Ernest Dichter: motive interpreter. *Journal of Advertising Research, 17*(3), 3–8.

Bauer, M. (1996). The narrative interview: Comments on a technique for qualitative data collection London School of Economics and Political Science. Methodology Institute. *Papers in Social Research Methods.*

Becker, G. S. & Murphy, K. M. (1988). A theory of rational addiction. *The Journal of Political Economy, 96*(4), 675–700.

Beenstock, M. & Rahav, G. (2002). Testing gateway theory: do cigarette prices affect illicit drug use? *Journal of Health Economics, 21*(4), 679–698.

Benedek, T. (1936). Dominant ideas and their relation to morbid cravings. *The International Journal of Psychoanalysis, 17*, 40.

Berent, I. (1961). A ritualistic aspect of smoking. *American Imago, 18*(3), 305–309.

Bernays, E. L. (1928). *Propaganda.* H. Liveright.

Bickel, W. K. & Marsch, L. A. (2001). Toward a behavioural economic understanding of drug dependence: delay discounting processes. *Addiction, 96*(1), 73–86.

Bion, W. R. (1959). Attacks on linking. *International Journal of Psychoanalysis 40*, 308–315.

Bion, W. R. (1977). *The seven servants.* Jason Aronson.

Blaszczynski, A. & Nower, L. (2002). A pathways model of problem and pathological gambling. *Addiction, 97* (5), 487–499.

Bollas, C. (1979). The transformational object. *The International Journal of Psychoanalysis, 60,* 97.

Bornstein, R. F. (1996). Beyond orality: toward an object relations/interactionist reconceptualization of the aetiology and dynamics of dependency. *Psychoanalytic Psychology, 13*(2), 177.

Bradley, B., Field, M., Mogg, K. & De Houwer, J. (2004). Attentional and evaluative biases for smoking cues in nicotine dependence: component processes of biases in visual orienting. *Behavioural Pharmacology, 15*(1), 29–36.

Bram, A. D., & Gabbard, G. O. (2001). Potential space and reflective functioning: towards conceptual clarification and preliminary clinical implications. *The International Journal of Psychoanalysis, 82*(4), 685–699.

Brill, A. A. (1922). Tobacco and the individual. *International Journal of Psycho-Analysis, 3,* 430–444.

British Psychological Society (2021). *Code of ethics and conduct.* https://doi.org/10.53841/bpsrep.2021.inf94

Brody, S. (1980). Transitional objects: idealization of a phenomenon. *The Psychoanalytic Quarterly, 49*(4), 561–605.

Brody, S. & Axelrad, S. (1970). *Anxiety and ego formation in infancy.* International Universities Press, Inc.

Brody, S. & Axelrad, S. (1978). *Mothers, fathers, and children. Explorations in the formation of character in the first seven years.* International Universities Press, Inc.

Burch, B. (1993). Gender identities, lesbianism, and potential space. *Psychoanalytic Psychology, 10*(3), 359.

Busch, F. (1974). Dimensions of the first transitional object. *The Psychoanalytic Study of the Child, 24,* 215–299.

Busch, F. & McKnight, J. (1973). Parental attitudes and the development of the primary transitional object. *Child Psychiatry and Human Development, 4,* 12–20.

Busch, F. & McKnight, J. (1977). Theme and variation in the development of the fist transitional object. *International Journal of Psychoanalysis, 58,* 479–486.

Busch, F. Nagera, H. McKnight, J. & Pezzarossi, G. (1973). Primary transitional objects. *Journal of the American Academy of Child Psychiatry, 12,* 183–214.

Cath, S. H. (1982). Adolescence and addiction to alternative belief systems: psychoanalytic and psychophysiological considerations. *Psychoanalytic Inquiry, 2*(4), 619–675.

Chatterji, A. (2009). 'Psychoanalysis and the unconscious' and D. W. Winnicott's transitional and related phenomena. *Psychoanalytic Review, 96*(5), 785–800.

Chen, X. G., Unger, J. B., Palmer, P., Weiner, M. D., Johnson, C. A., Wong, M. M. & Austin, G. (2002). Prior cigarette smoking initiation predicting current alcohol use: evidence for a gateway drug effect among California adolescents from eleven ethnic groups. *Addictive Behaviour, 27*(5), 799–817.

Childress, A. R., Ehrman, R., McLellan, A. T. & O'Brien, C. (1988). Conditioned craving and arousal in cocaine addiction: a preliminary report. *National Institute of Drug Abuse Research Monograph, 81,* 74–80.

Christiansen, B. A. & Goldman, M. S. (1983). Alcohol-related expectancies versus demographic / background variables in the prediction of adolescent drinking. *Journal of Consulting and Clinical Psychology, 51*(2), 249–257.

Civin, M., & Lombardi, K. L. (1990). The preconscious and potential space. *Psychoanalytic Review, 77*(4), 573.

Cloninger, C. R. (1987). A systematic method for clinical description and classification of personality variants. A proposal. *Archives of General Psychiatry, 44*(6), 573–588.

Cooper, S., & Adler, G. (1990). Toward a clarification of the transitional object and selfobject concepts in the treatment of the borderline patient. *The Annual of Psychoanalysis, 18*, 133–152.

Coppolillo, H. P. (1967). Maturational aspects of the transitional phenomenon. *The International Journal of Psychoanalysis, 48*(2), 237–246.

Corbin, J. & Strauss, S. (2008). *Basics of qualitative research: techniques and procedures for developing grounded theory.* (3rd ed). Sage Publications Ltd.

Coulthard, M., Farrell, M., Singleton, N., & Meltzer, H. (2002). *Tobacco, alcohol, and drug use and mental health.* Office for National Statistics. Retrieved 10 September 2017, from https://www.ons.gov.uk

Crowley, R. M. (1939). Psychoanalytic literature on drug addiction and alcoholism. *The Psychoanalytic Review (1913–1957), 26*, 39.

Davis, M. & Wallbridge, D. (1981). *Boundary and space: an introduction to the work of D. W. Winnicott.* Karnac Books.

Daniels, G. E. (1933). Clinical communications: turning points in the analysis of a case of alcoholism. *The Psychoanalytic Quarterly, 2*(1), 123–130.

Davidson, L. (1976). The transitional object in development and psychoanalysis (a symposium)—inanimate objects in psychoanalysis and their relation. *Contemporary Psychoanalysis, 12*, 479–488.

De Paula Ramos, S. (2004). What can we learn from psychoanalysis and prospective studies about chemically dependent patients? *International Journal of Psychoanalysis, 85*(2), 467–487.

Dichter, E. (1947). *The psychology of everyday living.* Barnes and Noble, Inc.

Dimen, M. (1991). Deconstructing difference: gender, splitting, and transitional space. *Psychoanalytic Dialogues, 1*(3), 335–352.

Dinnage, R. (1978). A bit of light. In S. Grolnick, L. Barkin, & W. Muensterberger (Eds.), *Between fantasy and reality: transitional objects and phenomena* (pp. 363–378). Jason Aronson.

Dithrich, C. W. (1991). Pseudologia fantastica, dissociation, and potential space, in child treatment. *The International Journal of Psychoanalysis, 72*(4), 657.

Dixon, M. R., Marley, J. & Jacobs, E. A. (2003). Delayed discounting by pathological gamblers. *Journal of Applied Behaviour Analysis, 36*(4), 449–458.

Dodes, L. M. (1990). Addiction, helplessness, and narcissistic rage. *The Psychoanalytic Quarterly, 59*(3), 398–419.

Dodes, L. M. (1996). Compulsion and addiction. *Journal of the American Psychoanalytic Association, 44*(3), 815–835.

Dodes, L. M. (2003). Addiction and psychoanalysis. *Canadian Journal of Psychoanalysis, 11*(1), 123.

Downey, T. W. (1978). Transitional phenomena in the analysis of early adolescent males. *The Psychoanalytic Study of the Child, 33*, 19–46.

Drummond, D. C. (2001). Theories of drug craving, ancient and modern. *Addiction, 96* (1), 33–46.

Drummond, D. C., Cooper, T. & Glautier, S. P. (1990). Conditioned learning in alcohol dependence: implications for cue exposure treatment. *British Journal of Addiction, 85*(6), 725–743.

Edwards, G. & Gross, M. M. (1976). Alcohol dependence: provisional description of a clinical syndrome. *British Medical Journal,* 1(6017), 1058–1061.

Ehrenberg, D. B. (1976). The "intimate edge" and the "third area". *Contemporary Psychoanalysis, 12*(4), 489–496.

Eigen, M. (1981). The area of faith in Winnicott, Lacan and Bion. *International Journal of Psychoanalysis, 62,* 413–33.

Einstein, S. & Epstein, A. (1980). Cigarette smoking contagion. *International Journal of the Addictions, 15*(1).

Elkind, S. N. (2002). Review essay on reading in a potential space. *Psychoanalytic Dialogues, 12*(2), 285–298.

Engel, J. F. (1961). Motivation research – magic or menace? *Michigan Business Review, 13,* 28–32.

Farrell, M., Howes, S., Bebbington, P., Brugha, T., Jenkins, R., Lewis, G., Marsden, J., Taylor, C. & Metzer, H. (2001). Nicotine, alcohol and drug dependence and psychiatric comorbidity: results of a national household survey. *The British Journal of Psychiatry, 179,* 432–437.

Ferrence, R. (2001). Diffusion theory and drug use. *Addiction,* 96(1), 165–173.

Fink, P. (1962). The pacifier as a transitional object. *Bulletin of the Philadelphia Association for Psychoanalysis, 12,* 69–83.

Fintzy, R. T. (1971). Vicissitudes of the transitional object in a borderline child. *The International Journal of Psychoanalysis, 52,* 107.

Fleming, M. (2005). The mental pain of the psychoanalyst: A personal view. *International Forum of Psychoanalysis, 14*(2), 69–75.

Freud, S. (1897). *The complete letters of Sigmund Freud to Wilhelm Fliess, 1887–1904.* Belknap Press.

Freud, S. (1898). Sexuality in the aetiology of the neuroses. In *The Standard Edition of the Complete Psychological Works of Sigmund Freud, Volume III: early psycho-analytic publications (1893–1899),* (pp. 263–286). Vintage Publishing.

Freud, S. (1910). 'Wild' psycho-analysis. In *The Standard Edition of the Complete Psychological Works of Sigmund Freud, Volume XI: five lectures on psycho-analysis, Leonardo da Vinci and other works (1910),* (pp. 219–228). Vintage Publishing.

Freud, S. (1914). Remembering, repeating and working through (further recommendations on the technique of psychoanalysis II). In *The Standard Edition of the Complete Psychological Works of Sigmund Freud, Volume XII: the case of Schreber, papers on technique and other works (1911–1913),* (pp. 147–156). Vintage Publishing.

Freud, S. (1927). The Future of an Illusion, In *The Standard Edition of the Complete Psychological Works of Sigmund Freud, Volume XXI: the future of an illusion, civilization and its discontents, and other works (1927–1931),* (pp. 1–56). Vintage Publishing.

Frosch, W. A. (1970). Psychoanalytic evaluation of addiction and habituation. *Journal of the American Psychoanalytic Association, 18*(1), 209–218.

Fullerton, R. A. (2005, May). The Devil's Lure? Motivation research, 1934–1954. In *Proceedings of the Conference on Historical Analysis and Research in Marketing* (Vol. 12, pp. 134–143).

Fullerton, R. A. (2013). The birth of consumer behavior: motivation research in the 1940s and 1950s. *Journal of Historical Research in Marketing, 5*(2), 212–222.

Gabbard, G. O. (2002). Addiction as mind-body bridge commentary on paper by Lisa Director. *Psychoanalytic Dialogues*, *12*(4), 581–584.

Gaddini, R. (2003). The precursors of transitional objects and phenomena. *Psychoanalysis and History*, *5*(1), 53–61.

Gaddini, R. & Gaddini, E. (1970). Transitional objects and the process of individuation: a study in three different social groups. *Journal of the American Academy of Child Psychiatry*, *9*, 347–365.

Gay, P. (1988). *Freud: A life for our time*. W. W. Norton & Company.

Gay, E. L. & Hyson, M. C. (1976). Blankets, bears, and bunnies: studies of children's contacts with treasured objects. In T. Shapiro (Ed.), *Psychoanalysis and contemporary science, vol. V* (pp. 271–316). International Universities Press, Inc.

Gelkopf, M., Levitt, S., & Bleich, A. (2002). An integration of three approaches to addiction and methadone maintenance treatment: the self-medication hypothesis, the disease model and social criticism. *Israel Journal of Psychiatry and Related Sciences*, *39*(2), 140.

Giovacchini, P. L. (1984). The psychoanalytic paradox: the self as a transitional object. *Psychoanalytic Review*, *71*(1), 81.

Giovacchini, P. (1987). The borderline state, the transitional object, and the psychoanalytic paradox. *The Borderline Patient*, *1*, 181–204.

Glaser, B. G., & Strauss, A. L. (1967). *The discovery of grounded theory: strategies for qualitative research*. Aldine Publishing Company.

Glover, E. (1932). On the aetiology of drug addiction. *The International Journal of Psychoanalysis*, *13*, 298.

Goldman, D. (1996). An exquisite corpse: The strain of working in and out of potential space. *Contemporary Psychoanalysis, 32*(3), 339–358.

Goldman, M. S., & Darkes, J. (2004). Alcohol expectancy multiaxial assessment: a memory network-based approach. *Psychological Assessment*, *16*(1), 4.

Gottdiener, W. H. (2006). A preliminary test of the addiction-to-near-death construct. *Psychoanalytic Psychology*, *23*(4), 661.

Grandy, M. A., & Tuber, S. (2009). Entry into imaginary space: metaphors of transition and variations in the affective quality of potential space in children's literature. *Psychoanalytic Psychology*, *26*(3), 274.

Green, G. H. (1923). Some notes on smoking. *The International Journal of Psycho-Analysis, 4*, 323.

Greenacre, P. (1969). The fetish and the transitional object. *The Psychoanalytic Study of the Child*, *24*(1), 144–164.

Greenacre, P. (1970). The transitional object and the fetish with special reference to the role of illusion. *The International Journal of Psychoanalysis*, *51*, 447.

Greenson, R. R. (1954). About the sound 'Mm…'. *The Psychoanalytic Quarterly*, *23*(2), 234–239.

Grolnick, S. & Lengyel, A. (1978). Etruscan burial symbols and the transitional process. In S. Grolnick, L. Barkin, & W. Muensterberger (Eds.), *Between fantasy and reality: transitional objects and phenomena* (pp. 379–410). Jason Aronson.

Gwaltney, C. J., Shiffman, S., Norman, G. J., Paty, J. A., Kassel, J. D., Gnys, M., Hickcox, M., Waters, A. & Balabanis, M. (2001). Does smoking abstinence self-efficacy vary across situations? Identifying context-specificity within the Relapse Situation Efficacy Questionnaire. *Journal of Consulting and Clinical Psychology*, *69*(3), 516–527.

Haaken, J. (1992) Beyond addiction: recovery groups and 'women who love too much'. *Free Associations*, *3*, 85–109.

Haire, M. (1950). Projective techniques in marketing research. *Journal of Marketing, 14*(5), 649–656.

Hanchett, S., & Casale, L. (1976). The theory of transitional phenomena and cultural symbols. *Contemporary Psychoanalysis, 12*(4), 496–507.

Harper, D. (2022). Addiction. In *Online Etymology Dictionary*. Retrieved 27 January 2023, from https://www.etymonline.com/word/addiction#etymonline_v_25996

Harris, H. I. (1964). Gambling addiction in an adolescent male. *The Psychoanalytic Quarterly, 33*(4), 513–525.

Henry, W. E. (1947). Art and cultural symbolism: a psychological study of greeting cards. *Journal of Aesthetics and Art Criticism [Online]. 6*(1), 36–44.

Hiller, E. (1922). Some remarks on tobacco. *International Journal of Psycho-Analysis, 3,* 475–480.

Hinshelwood, R. D. (1991). *A dictionary of Kleinian thought* (2nd ed.). Free Association Books.

Hinshelwood, R. D. (2013). *Research on the couch: single case studies, subjectivity, and psychoanalytic knowledge.* Routledge.

Hollway, W., & Jefferson, T. (1997). Eliciting narrative through the in-depth interview. *Qualitative Inquiry, 3*(1), 53–70.

Hollway, W. & Jefferson, T. (2013). *Doing qualitative research differently: a psychosocial approach* (2nd ed.). Sage Publications Ltd.

Hong, K. M. (1978). The transitional phenomena. A theoretical integration. *The psychoanalytic study of the child, 33,* 47–79.

Hong, K. M. & Townes, B. D. (1976). Infants' attachment to inanimate objects: a cross-cultural study. *Journal of the American Academy of Child Psychiatry, 15,* 49–61.

Hopkins, B. (2002). 'Every man kills the thing he loves': object-use and potential space in *The Winter's Tale. The Psychoanalytic Review, 89*(2), 195–216.

Hopper, E. (1995). A psychoanalytical theory of drug addiction: unconscious fantasies of homosexuality, compulsions and masturbation within the context of traumatogenic processes. *International Journal of Psycho-Analysis, 76*(6), 1121–1142.

Horowitz, D. (1986). *The birth of a salesman: Ernest Dichter and the objects of desire* (vol. 83). Daniel Horowitz.

Horton, P. C. (1977). Personality disorder and hard-to-diagnose schizophrenia. *Journal of Operational Psychiatry, 8,* 70–81.

Horton, P. C., Louy, J. W. & Coppolillo, H. P. (1974). Personality disorder and transitional relatedness. *Archives of General Psychiatry, 30,* 618–622.

Jacobs, M. (1995). *D. W. Winnicott*. Sage Publications.

Jacobson, L. (2003). On the use of 'sexual addiction': the case for 'perversion'. *Contemporary Psychoanalysis, 39*(1), 107–113.

Jemstedt, A. (2000, January). Potential space – the place of encounter between inner and outer reality. *International Forum of Psychoanalysis, 9*(1–2), 124–131.

Johnson, B. (1999). Three perspectives on addiction. *Journal of the American Psychoanalytic Association, 47*(3), 791–815.

Johnson, B. (2003). Psychological addiction, physical addiction, addictive character, and addictive personality disorder: a nosology of addictive disorders. *Canadian Journal of Psychoanalysis, 11,* 135–160.

Jones, A. M. (1989). A systems approach to the demand for alcohol and tobacco. *Bulletin of Economic Research, 41*(2), 85–105.

Jones, E. (1972). Chapter XIII. The Fliess Period (1887–1902). In *Sigmund Freud: Life and Work, Volume One: The Young Freud 1856–1900 Volume 45* (pp. 316–350). Basic Books Publishing Co., Inc.

Joseph, B. (1982). Addiction to near-death. *International Journal of Psychoanalysis 63*, 449–456.

Jovchelovitch, S., & Bauer, M. W. (2000). Narrative interviewing. *Qualitative Researching with Text, Image and Sound, 57*, 74.

Kafka, J. S. (1969). The body as transitional object: a psychoanalytic study of a self-mutilating patient. *British Journal of Medical Psychology, 42*(3), 207–212.

Kahne, M. J. (1967). On the persistence of transitional phenomena into adult life. *The International Journal of Psychoanalysis*, 48, 247–258.

Kandel, D. B., Yamaguchi, K. & Chen, K. (1992). Stages of progression in drug involvement from adolescence to adulthood: further evidence for the gateway theory. *Journal of Studies in Alcohol, 53*(5).

Kearney, M. H. & O'Sullivan, J. (2003). Identity shifts as turning points in health behaviour change. *Western Journal of Nursing Research, 25*(2), 134–152.

Keiser, S. (1948). The psychology of everyday living. *Psychoanalytic Quarterly, 17*, 284.

Kenkel, D., Mathios, A. D. & Pacula, R. L. (2001). Economics of youth drug use, addiction and gateway effects. *Addiction, 96*(1), 151–164.

Khantzian, E. J. (1978). The ego, the self and opiate addiction: theoretical and treatment considerations. *International Review of Psycho-Analysis*.

Khantzian, E. J. (1987). The self-medication hypothesis of addictive disorders: focus on heroin and cocaine dependence. *The Cocaine Crisis*, 65–74.

Khantzian, E. J. (1997). The self-medication hypothesis of substance use disorders: a reconsideration and recent applications. *Harvard Review of Psychiatry, 4*(5).

Khantzian, E. J. (2005). New windows on understanding addictive vulnerability: commentary on papers by Lisa Director and Noelle Burton. *Psychoanalytic Dialogues, 15*(4), 613–619.

Klein, M. (1946). Notes on Some Schizoid Mechanisms. *International Journal of Psychoanalysis, 27*, 99–110.

Klein, M. (1975). *Envy and gratitude and other works 1946–1963*. The Free Press.

Knafo, D. (2008). The senses grow skilled in their craving: thoughts on creativity and addiction. *The Psychoanalytic Review, 95*(4), 571–595.

Kohut, H. (1971). *The analysis of the self: a systematic approach to the psychoanalytic treatment of narcissistic personality disorders*. University of Chicago Press.

Kuhn, T. S. (1962). *The structure of scientific revolutions*. University of Chicago Press.

Kuriloff, E. (1998). Winnicott and Sullivan: playing with the interpersonal model in a transitional space. *Contemporary Psychoanalysis, 34*(3), 379–388.

LaMothe, R. (2005). Creating space: the fourfold dynamics of potential space. *Psychoanalytic Psychology, 22*(2), 207.

Lane, R. C., Hull, J. W., & Foehrenbach, L. M. (1991). The addiction to negativity. *Psychoanalytic Review, 78*(3), 391.

Lazarsfeld, P. F. (1937). The use of detailed interviews in market research. *Journal of Marketing, 2*(1), 3–8.

Levy, S. (2003). Roots of marketing and consumer research at the University of Chicago. *Consumption, Markets and Culture 6*(2), 99–110.

Levy, S. (2005). The evolution of qualitative research in marketing. *Journal of Business Research 58*(3), 341–347.

Lewis, M. J. (1990). Alcohol: mechanisms of addiction and reinforcement. *Advances in Alcohol & Substance Abuse*, *9*(1–2), 47–66.

Lewit, E. M. (1989). U.S. tobacco taxes: behavioural effects and policy implications. *British Journal of Addiction*, *84*(10), 1217–1234.

Lindsay, G. B. & Rainey, J. (1997). Psychosocial and pharmacologic explanations of nicotine's 'gateway drug' function. *Journal of School Health*, *67*(4), 123–126.

Lindzey, G. (1952). Thematic appreciation test: interpretive assumptions and related empirical evidence. *Psychological Bulletin*, *49*(1), 1–25.

Lubman, D. I., Yücel, M. & Pantelis, C. (2004). Addiction, a condition of compulsive behaviour? Neuroimaging and neuropsychological evidence of inhibitory dysregulation. *Addiction*, *99*(12), 1491–1502.

McDonald, M. (1970). Transitional tunes and musical development. *The Psychoanalytic Study of the Child*, *25*, 215–299.

Madden, G. J., Bickel, W. K., & Jacobs, E. A. (1999). Discounting of delayed rewards in opioid-dependent outpatients: exponential or hyperbolic discounting functions? *Experimental and Clinical Psychopharmacology*, *7*(3), 284.

Madden, G. J., Petry, N. M., Badger, G. J., & Bickel, W. K. (1997). Impulsive and self-control choices in opioid-dependent patients and non-drug-using control patients: Drug and monetary rewards. *Experimental and Clinical Psychopharmacology*, *5*(3), 256.

Malinowska D. (2018). How to counter the ten myths about work addiction? Three postulates for future research. *Journal of Behavioural Addictions*, *7*(4), 871–874.

Mann, G. (1998). From disintegration to unintegration: the creation of potential space through work with dreams. *Journal of the American Academy of Psychoanalysis*, *26*(3), 389–416.

Marcovitz, E. (1969). On the nature of addiction to cigarettes. *Journal of the American Psychoanalytic Association*, *17*(4), 1074–1096.

Marlatt, G. A. (1979). A cognitive-behavioural model of the relapse process. *National Institute on Drug Abuse Research Monograph*, *25*, 191–200.

Marlatt, G. A. (1996). Taxonomy of high-risk situations for alcohol relapse: evolution and development of a cognitive-behavioural model. *Addiction*, *91* (Supp.), S37–S49.

Melchior, C. L., & Tabakoff, B. (1984). A conditioning model of alcohol tolerance. *Recent Developments in Alcoholism: Volume 2*, 5–16.

Meltzer, H. (1996). *Economic activity and social functioning of residents with psychiatric disorders.* OPCS Surveys of Psychiatric Morbidity in Great Britain Report no.3. HMSO.

Menninger, K. A. (1934). Polysurgery and polysurgical addiction. *The Psychoanalytic Quarterly*, *3*(2), 173–199.

Menzies Lyth, I., & Trist, E. (1989). Pleasure foods, In I. Menzies Lyth, *The dynamics of the social: selected essays vol. II* (pp. 68–89). Free Association Books.

Miller, J. (2002). Heroin addiction: the needle as transitional object. *Journal of the American Academy of Psychoanalysis and Dynamic Psychiatry*, *30*(2), 293–304.

Miller, M. C. (1992). Winnicott unbound: The fiction of Philip Roth and the sharing of potential space. *International Review of Psycho-Analysis*, *19*, 445–456.

Miller, P. & Rose, N. (1997). Mobilising the consumer: assembling the subject of consumption. *Theory, Culture and Society*, *14*(1), 1–36.

Milner, M. (1952). Aspects of symbolism in comprehension of the not-self. *International Review of Psychoanalysis*, *33*, 181–194.

Modell, A. H. (1963). Primitive object relationships and the pre-disposition to schizophrenia. *The International Journal of Psychoanalysis*, *44*, 282.

Modell, A. H. (1970). The transitional object and the creative act. *The Psychoanalytic Quarterly*, *39*(2), 240–250.

Nelson, M. R. (2007). The hidden persuaders. *Journal of Advertising*, *37*(1), 113–126.

Niaura, R. (2000). Cognitive social learning and related perspectives on drug craving. *Addiction*, *95*(8s2), 155–163.

O'Brien, C. P., Childress, A. R., McLellan, A. T., & Ehrman, R. (1992). A learning model of addiction. *Research Publications – Association for Research in Nervous and Mental Disease*, 70, 157–177.

O'Brien, M., Singleton, N., Sparks, J., Meltzer, H., & Brugha, T. (2002). *Adults with a psychotic disorder living in private households, 2000*. The Stationery Office.

Ogden, T. H. (1985). On potential space. *International Review of Psychoanalysis*, *66*, 129–141.

Oral Cancer Foundation (2010).

Orford, J. (2001). Addiction as an excessive appetite. *Addiction*, *96*(1), 15–31.

Os, M. (1991). Observations on the formation and function of a transitional object: Stages in internalisation. *The Scandinavian psychoanalytic review*, *14*(1), 1–18.

Oxford University Press (n.d.). Addiction. In *Oxford Learner's Dictionary*. Retrieved 29 July 2023, https://www.oxfordlearnersdictionaries.com/definition/english/addiction?q=addiction

Packard, V. (1957). *The hidden persuaders* (2nd ed.). Ig Publishing.

Parker, C. (1979). *Mother-infant interactions and infants' use of transitional objects*. Dissertation, Columbia University.

Parrish, D. (1978). Transitional objects and phenomena in a case of twinship. In S. Grolnick, L. Barkin, & W. Muensterberger (Eds.), *Between fantasy and reality: transitional objects and phenomena* (pp. 271–287). Jason Aronson.

Paskauskas, R. A. (Ed.). (1993). *The complete correspondence of Sigmund Freud and Ernest Jones, 1909–1939*. Belknap Press.

Pedder, J. (1992). Conductor or director? Transitional space in psychotherapy and in the theater. *Psychoanalytic Review*, *79*(2), 261–270.

Phillips, A. (1988). *Winnicott*. Fontana.

Pizer, S. A. (1996). Negotiating potential space illusion, play, metaphor, and the subjunctive. *Psychoanalytic Dialogues*, *6*(5), 689–712.

Politz, A. (1956). 'Motivation research' from a research viewpoint. *The Public Opinion Quarterly*, *20*(4), 663–673.

Pritchard, W. S., Robinson, J. H., Guy, T. D., Davis, R. A., & Stiles, M. F. (1996). Assessing the sensory role of nicotine in cigarette smoking. *Psychopharmacology*, *127*, 55–62.

Prochaska, J. O., DiClemente, C. C., Velicer, W. F., Ginpil, S. & Norcross, J. C. (1985). Predicting change in smoking status for self-changers. *Addictive Behaviours*, *10*(4), 395–406.

Prochaska, J. O., & Goldstein, M. G. (1991). Process of smoking cessation: implications for clinicians. *Clinics in Chest Medicine*, *12*(4), 727–735.

Prochoska, J. O., & Velicer, W. F. (1997). The transtheoretical model of health behaviour change. *American Journal of Health Promotion*, *12*, 38–48.

Provence, S. & Lipton, R. C. (1962). *Infants in institutions. A comparison of their development with family-reared infants during the first year of life*. International Universities Press, Inc.

Radó, S. (1926). The psychic effects of intoxicants: an attempt to evolve a psycho-analytical theory of morbid cravings. *The International Journal of Psychoanalysis*, *7*, 396.

Radó, S. (1928). The psychical effects of intoxication. *The International Journal of Psychoanalysis*, *9*, 301.

Radó, S. (1933). The psychoanalysis of pharmacothymia (drug addiction). *The Psychoanalytic Quarterly*, *2*(1), 1–23.

Rather, B. C., Goldman, M. S., Roehrich, L. & Brannick, M. (1992). Empirical modelling of an alcohol expectancy memory network using multidimensional scaling. *Journal of Abnormal Psychology*, *101*(1), 174–183.

Resch, R. C., Pizzuti, S., & Woods, A. (1988). The later creation of a transitional object. *Psychoanalytic psychology*, *5*(4), 369.

Riggall, R. M. (1923). Homosexuality and alcoholism. *The Psychoanalytic Review (1913–1957)*, *10*, 157.

Robbins, B. S. (1935). A note on the significance of infantile nutritional disturbances in the development of alcoholism. *The Psychoanalytic Review (1913–1957)*, *22*, 53.

Robinson, T. E. & Berridge, K. C. (1993). The neural basis of drug craving: an incentive-sensitization theory of addiction. *Brain Research Reviews*, *18*(3), 247–291.

Robinson, T. E. & Berridge, K. C. (2003). Addiction. *Annual Review of Psychology*, *54*(1), 25–53.

Rodman, F. R. (1987). *The spontaneous gesture: selected letters of D. W. Winnicott.* Harvard University Press.

Roiphe, H., & Galenson, E. (1975). Some observations on transitional object and infantile fetish. *The Psychoanalytic Quarterly*, *44*(2), 206–231.

Rosenfeld, H. A. (1960). On drug addiction. *International Journal of Psychoanalysis*, *41*, 467–475.

Rosenthal, G. (1993). Reconstruction of life stories: principles of selection in generating stories for narrative biographical interviews. *The Narrative Study of Lives*, *1*(1), 59–91.

Rothwell, N. D. (1955). Motivational research revisited. *Journal of Marketing*, *20*(2), 150–154.

Rycroft, C. (1985). *Psychoanalysis and Beyond.* Hogarth Press.

Samuel, L. R. (2010). *Freud on Madison Avenue: motivation research and subliminal advertising in America.* University of Pennsylvania Press.

Samuels, A. (1993). *The political psyche.* Routledge.

Savitt, R. A. (1963). Psychoanalytic studies on addiction: ego structure in narcotic addiction. *The Psychoanalytic Quarterly*, *32*(1), 43–57.

Schlierf, C. (1983). Transitional objects and object relationship in a case of anxiety neurosis. *International Review of Psychoanalysis*, *10*(3), 319–332.

Schulteis, G., & Koob, G. F. (1996). Reinforcement processes in opiate addiction: a homeostatic model. *Neurochemical Research*, *21*, 1437–1454.

Schur, E. M. (1963). *Narcotic addiction in Britain and America*, 69–164.

Schütze, F. (1992a). Pressure and guilt: war experiences of a young German soldier and their biographical implications (part 1). *International Sociology*, *7*(2), 187–208.

Schütze, F. (1992b). Pressure and guilt: war experiences of a young German soldier and their biographical implications (part 2). *International Sociology*, *7*(3), 347–367.

Scott, A. (2018). *The centrality of research: A BPC policy document.* British Psychoanalytic Council. https://www.bpc.org.uk/download/487/BPC-The-Centrality-of-Research.pdf

Segal, J. (1992). *Key figures in counselling and psychotherapy: Melanie Klein.* Sage Publications.

Siegel, S. & Ramos, B. M. (2002). Applying laboratory research: drug anticipation and the treatment of drug addiction. *Experimental and Clinical Psychopharmacology*, *10*(3), 162–183.

Simmel, E. (1948). Alcoholism and addiction. *The Psychoanalytic Quarterly*, *17*(1), 6–31.

Skog, O. J. (2000). Addicts' choice. *Addiction*, *95*(9), 1309–1314.

Sloate, P. L. (2008). From fetish object to transitional object: the analysis of a chronically self-mutilating bulimic patient. *Journal of the American Academy of Psychoanalysis and Dynamic Psychiatry, 36*(1), 69–88.

Slovic, P. M., Finucane, M., Peters, E. & MacGregor, D. G. (2006). The affect heuristic. *European Journal of Operational Research, 177*(3), 1333–1352.

Smith, J. A. (2008). *Qualitative psychology: a practical guide to research methods* (2nd ed.). Sage Publications Ltd.

Smith, J. A., Flowers, P. & Larkin, M. (2009). *Interpretative phenomenological analysis: theory, method and research.* Sage Publications Ltd.

Solomon, R. L. (1980). The opponent-process theory of acquired motivation: the costs of pleasure and the benefits of pain. *American Psychology, 35*(8), 691–712.

Solomon, R. L. & Corbit, J. D. (1973). An opponent-process theory of motivation: II. Cigarette addiction. *Journal of Abnormal Psychology, 81*(2), 158–171.

Sonnenfeld, J. A. (1985). Shedding light on the Hawthorne studies. *Journal of Occupational Behaviour, 6*(2), 111–130.

Stern, B. (2004). The importance of being Ernest: commemorating Ditcher's contribution to advertising research. *Journal of Advertising Research, 44*(2), 165–169.

Stevenson, O., & Winnicott, D. W. (1954). The first treasured possession: A study of the part played by specially loved objects and toys in the lives of certain children. *The Psychoanalytic Study of the Child, 9*(1), 199–217.

Straetz, M. R. (1976). Transitional phenomena in the treatment of adolescents. *Contemporary Psychoanalysis, 12*(4), 507–513.

Sugarman, A., & Kurash, C. (1982a). The body as a transitional object in bulimia. *International Journal of Eating Disorders, 1*(4), 57–67.

Sugarman, A., & Kurash, C. (1982b). Marijuana abuse, transitional experience, and the borderline adolescent. *Psychoanalytic Inquiry, 2*(4), 519–538.

Summers, F. (1999). Psychoanalytic boundaries and transitional space. *Psychoanalytic Psychology, 16*(1), 3.

Szasz, T. S. (1958). The role of the counterphobic mechanism in addiction. *Journal of the American Psychoanalytic Association, 6*(2), 309–325.

Tadajewski, M. (2006). Remembering motivation research: toward an alternative genealogy of interpretive consumer research. *Marketing Theory, 6*(4), 429–466.

Tate, J. C., Stanton, A. L., Green, S. B., Schmitz, J. M., Le, T. & Marshall, B. (1994). Experimental analysis of the role of expectancy in nicotine withdrawal. *Psychology of Addictive Behaviours, 8*(3), 169–178.

The Tavistock and Portman NHS Foundation Trust. (2018). *Tavistock Adult Depression Study (TADS).* https://tavistockandportman.nhs.uk/research-and-innovation/our-research/research-projects/tavistock-adult-depression-study-tads/

Teitelbaum, S. (2003). Playing with Winnicott: A patient's account of her experience using the analyst as a transitional object. *Canadian Journal of Psychoanalysis, 11*(2), 435.

Tibon, S. (2005). On potential space in psychosomatics and psychosis: a Rorschach study. *Journal of the American Psychoanalytic Association, 1296–8.*

Tiffany, S. T. (1990). A cognitive model of drug urges and drug-use behaviour: role of automatic and non-automatic processes. *Psychological Review, 97*(2), 147–168.

Tiffany, S. T. (1999). Cognitive concepts of craving. *Alcohol Research and Health, 23*(3), 51–62.

Tiffany, S. T., & Conklin, C. A. (2000). A cognitive processing model of alcohol craving and compulsive alcohol use. *Addiction, 95*(8s2), 145–153.

Tolpin, M. (1971). On the beginnings of a cohesive self: an application of the concept of transmuting internalization to the study of the transitional object and signal anxiety. *The Psychoanalytic Study of the Child*, *26*(1), 316–352.

Torches of Freedom Campaign (n.d). *Torches of Freedom Campaign · American Women in Tobacco Advertisements 1929–1939 · Digital History - Histoire Numérique*. Retrieved 19 October 2023, from https://biblio.uottawa.ca/omeka2/jmccutcheon/exhibits/show/american-women-in-tobacco-adve/torches-of-freedom-campaign

Tullis, L. M., Dupont, R., Frost-Pineda, K., & Gold, M. S. (2003). Marijuana and tobacco: a major connection? *Journal of Addictive Diseases*, *22*(3), 51–62.

Turkel, A. R. (1998). All about Barbie: distortions of a transitional object. *Journal of the American Academy of Psychoanalysis*, *26*(1), 165–177.

Ulman, R. B., & Paul, H. (2013). *The self psychology of addiction and its treatment: Narcissus in wonderland*. Routledge.

United States Department of Health, Education, and Welfare: Public Health Service (1964). *Smoking and Health: Report of the Advisory Committee to the Surgeon General of the Public Health Service*. https://www.govinfo.gov/content/pkg/GPO-SMOKINGANDHEALTH/pdf/GPO-SMOKINGANDHEALTH.pdf

Usuelli, A. K. (1972). The significance of illusion in the work of Freud and Winnicott: a controversial issue. *International Review of Psychoanalysis*, *19*, 179–187.

Vivona, J. M. (2000). Toward autonomous desire: women's worry as post-oedipal transitional object. *Psychoanalytic Psychology*, *17*(2), 243.

Volkan, V. D. & Kavanaugh, J. G. (1978). The cat people. In S. Grolnick, L. Barkin, & W. Muensterberger (Eds.), *Between fantasy and reality: transitional objects and phenomena* (pp. 289–303). Jason Aronson.

Vygotsky, L. S. (1967). Play and its role in the mental development of the child. *Soviet Psychology*, *5*(3), 6–18.

Waters, A. J. & Feyerabend, C. (2000). Determinants and effects of attentional bias in smokers. *Psychology of Addictive Behaviours*, *14*(2), 111–120.

Waters, A. J., Shiffman, S., Bradley, B. P. & Mogg, K. (2003). Attentional shifts to smoking cues in smokers. *Addiction*, *98*(10), 1409–1417.

West, R. (2006). *Theory of addiction*. Blackwell Publishing Ltd.

White, N. M. (1996). Addictive drugs as reinforcers: multiple partial actions on memory systems. *Addiction*, *91*(7), 921–949.

Wieder, H., & Kaplan, E. H. (1969). Drug use in adolescents – psychodynamic meaning and pharmacogenic effect. *Psychoanalytic Study of the Child*, *24*, 399–431.

Williams, R. J. (1957). Is it true what they say about motivation research? *Journal of Marketing*, *22*(2), 125–133.

Winick, C. (1955). *Trends in human relations research: the Sigmund Livingston fellowship program*. Anti-defamation League of B'nai B'rith.

Winnicott, D. W. (1945). Towards and objective study of human nature. In L. Caldwell & H. Taylor Robinson (Eds.), (2016), *The collected works of D. W. Winnicott: Volume 2, 1939–1945*. Oxford Academic. https://doi.org/10.1093/med:psych/9780190271343.003.0061

Winnicott, D. W. (1949). Hate in the counter-transference. *International Journal of Psychoanalysis*, *30*, 69–74.

Winnicott, D. W. (1950). 'Yes, but how do we know it's true?' In L. Caldwell & H. Taylor Robinson (Eds.), (2016), *The collected works of D. W. Winnicott: Volume 3, 1946–1951*. Oxford Academic. https://doi.org/10.1093/med:psych/9780190271350.003.0082

Winnicott, D. W. (1951). Transitional objects and transitional phenomena. In L. Caldwell & H. Taylor Robinson (Eds.), (2016), *The collected works of D. W.*

Winnicott: Volume 3, 1946–1951. Oxford Academic. https://doi.org/10.1093/med:ps ych/9780190271350.003.0088

Winnicott, D. W. (1953). Transitional objects and transitional phenomena – a study of the first not-me possession. *International Journal of Psychoanalysis, 34,* 89–97.

Winnicott, D. W. (1955a). Group influences and the maladjusted child: the school aspect. In L. Caldwell & H. Taylor Robinson (Eds.), (2016), *The collected works of D. W. Winnicott: Volume 5, 1955–1959.* Oxford Academic. https://doi.org/10.1093/med:psych/9780190271374.003.0009

Winnicott, D. W. (1955b). Letter to Charles M. Schulz. In L. Caldwell & H. Taylor Robinson (Eds.), (2016), *The collected works of D. W. Winnicott: Volume 5, 1955–1959.* Oxford Academic. https://doi.org/10.1093/med:psych/9780190271374.003.0022

Winnicott, D. W. (1956). The antisocial tendency. In L. Caldwell & H. Taylor Robinson (Eds.), (2016), *The collected works of D. W. Winnicott: Volume 5, 1955–1959.* Oxford Academic. https://doi.org/10.1093/med:psych/9780190271374.003.0031

Winnicott, D. W. (1958). Primary maternal preoccupation. In L. Caldwell & H. Taylor Robinson (Eds.), (2016), *The collected works of D. W. Winnicott: Volume 5, 1955–1959.* Oxford Academic. https://doi.org/10.1093/med:psych/9780190271374.003.0039

Winnicott, D. W. (1960). The theory of the parent-infant relationship. *International Journal of Psychoanalysis, 41,* 585–595.

Winnicott, D. W. (1964). *The child, the family and the outside world.* Penguin Books.

Winnicott, D. W. (1965a). *The family and individual development.* Tavistock Publications.

Winnicott, D. W. (1965b). *The maturational process and the facilitating environment: studies in the theory of emotional development.* Hogarth Press.

Winnicott, D. W. (1971a). *Playing and reality.* Routledge.

Winnicott, D. W. (1971b). *Therapeutic consultations in child psychiatry.* Basic Books.

Winnicott, D. W. (1975). *Collected papers: through paediatrics to psychoanalysis.* Tavistock Publications.

Winnicott, D. W. (1984). Comments on the report of the committee on punishment in prisons and borstals. In L. Caldwell & H. Taylor Robinson (Eds.), (2016), *The collected works of D. W. Winnicott: Volume 6, 1960–1963.* Oxford Academic. https://doi.org/10.1093/med:psych/9780190271381.003.0045

Winnicott, D. W. (1986). *Home is where we start from: essays by a psychoanalyst.* Penguin Books.

Winnicott, D. W. (1988a). *Babies and their mothers.* Free Association Books.

Winnicott, D. W. (1988b). *Human nature.* Free Association Books.

Woodman, M. (1982). *Addiction to perfection: the still unravished bride, a psychological study.* Inner City Books.

Woodward, J. L., Hofler, D., Haviland, F., Peterman, J., & Rosten, H. (1950). Depth interviewing. *Journal of Marketing, 14*(5), 721–724.

Woollcott, P. (1981). Addiction: clinical and theoretical considerations. *Annual of Psychoanalysis, 9,* 189–204.

World Health Organization. (2010). *Lexicon of alcohol and drug terms published by the World Health Organization.* Retrieved 5 July 2010, from http://www.who.int/substance_abuse/terminology/who_lexicon/en/

World Health Organization. (2022). *Tobacco.* https://www.who.int/news-room/fact-sheets/detail/tobacco

Zinberg, N. E. (1975). Addiction and ego function. *The Psychoanalytic Study of the Child, 30*(1), 567–588.

Index

Note: **Bold** page numbers indicate tables.

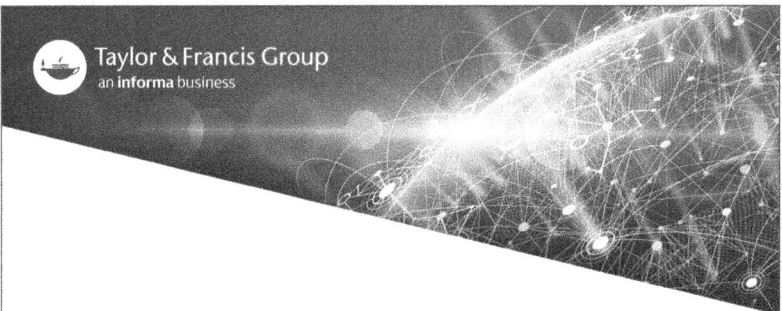
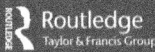
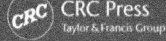